Kipaitapiiwahsinnooni [1]

Alcohol and Drug Abuse Education Program

Makai'stoo
Leo Fox

STANDINGALONE
Niitsitapoiyi
2000

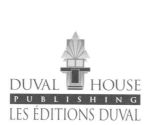

DUVAL HOUSE
PUBLISHING
LES ÉDITIONS DUVAL

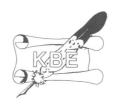

Printed in Canada. 5   4   3   2   1

Duval House Publishing/Les Éditions Duval, Inc.

Head Office
18228 - 102 Avenue
Edmonton, Alberta
CANADA T5S 1S7
Telephone: 1-800-267-6187
Fax: (780) 482-7213
e-mail: pdr@compusmart.ab.ca
website: www.duvalhouse.com

Ontario Office
5 Graham Avenue
Ottawa, Ontario
CANADA K1S 0B6

Kainaiwa Board of Education
P.O. Box 240
Standoff, Alberta
CANADA T0L 1Y0
Telephone: (403) 737-3966
Fax: (403) 737-2361

National Library of Canada Cataloguing in Publication Data

Fox, Leo.
  Kipaitapiiwahsinnooni

  Copublished by: Kainaiwa Board of Education.
  ISBN 1-55220-219-4

  1. Kainai Indians—Study and teaching (Secondary) 3. Alcoholism—Study and teaching (Secondary) 3. Drug abuse—Study and teaching (Secondary) I. Kainaiwa Board of Education. II. Title. III. Title: Alcohol and drug abuse program.
E99.K15F69 2001   971.23'004973   C2001-910704-8

 Kainaiwa Board of Education would like to acknowledge the financial support of the Aboriginal Healing Foundation.

Canadä We acknowledge the financial support of the Government of Canada through the Book Publishing Industry Development Program (BPIDP) for our publishing activities.

Photo Credits

- Allen Wells
  pp. 2, 4, 20, 24, 36, 40, 42, 45, 58, 60, 66, 101, 104, 121
- PROVINCIAL ARCHIVES OF ALBERTA
  pp. 10, 13, 31, 33, 47, 49, 52, 71, 77, 82, 87, 89, 93, 113
- Mrs. Josephine Soop
  pp. 8, 75, bottom back cover
- Sir Alexander Galt Museum and Archives
  p. 107, top and center back cover
- Henry Standing Alone
  cover

Acknowledgements

The research and publication for this curriculum was made possible by a grant from the federal government's Aboriginal Healing Foundation, Ottawa.

To Kainai Board of Education members for encouraging the development of this curriculum: Arnold Fox, Narcisse Blood, Richard Mills, Robert Calf, Toby Goodstriker, Winston Day Chief Jr. and Barney Day Chief.

The Blood First Nation elders especially: Adam Delany, Rufus Goodstriker, Bill Heavy Runner, Rosie Red Crow, Rosie Day Rider, Louise Crop Eared Wolf, Rachel Crying Head and Irene Day Rider for sharing their knowledge and wisdom.

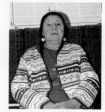

Kainai elder Rosie Day Rider is also known by her Blackfoot name Taakiohsin. She is a past member of the Mao'to'kiiksi, one of the sacred societies of Kainai. She was the main bundle holder for a number of the years that she was an active member. Through the teachings of her father, Aimmoniisi(Laurie Plume), and her involvement in Kainai traditional culture, she is a storehouse of traditional knowledge and a valuable resource for this project. Rosie continues to serve as a grandmother to the Mao'to'kiiksi. She is also much sought after as a face-painter.

Rosie had to raise her 10 children almost single-handedly after her late husband was crippled in an automobile accident. Because of this, she is just as experienced in dealing with contemporary matters as she is in talking about Kainai spirituality, culture, and history.

To residential school survivors who shared their experiences. To Alberta Provincial Archives for use of their photographs. To the Galt Museum Archives for use of their photographs. To Kainai First Nation members: Mrs. Josephine Soop, Mr. Wilfred Soop, Gordon and Loretta Manyfingers, Debbie Wells and Louis Soop for use of their photographs.

To the artists: Allen Wells for the illustrations and Henry Standing Alone for the cover design.

Message from the Kainai Board of Education Superintendent of Schools

Oki! I am very honoured to address the audience who will be learning from the *Kipaitapiiwahsinnooni* curriculum. It has been written primarily for the students of the Kainai High School. It is anticipated, however, that other First Nation schools and perhaps some public schools with native students will also use it.

The Healing Foundation funded this curriculum. As such, it addresses some of the inter-generational effects of the residential school era. Through interviews which are included in this curriculum, it is hoped that students will realize the root cause for much of the alcohol and drug abuse that exists among our people.

The writer of this series, Leo Fox, has focussed on creating an awareness of these abuse issues. More important, however, is the creation of a cultural and spiritual awareness that has been sadly lacking in many curriculum resources. This awareness will provide support for our young people.

Among the Kainai, we are very fortunate that we still have the elders who can provide us with their cultural and spiritual expertise. Their presence has kept our tribe intact. The sharing of their knowledge and their spirituality keeps alive a spiritual and cultural tradition which was targeted for extinction when the missionaries and colonial government agents first set foot on our land.

Young people, may the Creator guide you in all of your dreams and endeavours. Be strong and keep up your hopes in all that you pursue.

Joyce Goodstriker, B.Ed., Prof. Dip., M.Ed.
Superintendent of Education

TABLE OF CONTENTS

Introduction

Be Proud of Yourself: Know Who You Are

Oki. Nitsiitsitapiinihka'siim Makai'sto. Kakato'si, the late Dan Chief Moon gave me this name. It was my dad's father's name. It means "Wolf Crow." My English name is Leo Joseph Fox. I am the writer of this curriculum for our tribe. It is about alcohol and drug abuse education but it is also about our lives.

First of all, let me begin by telling you that I am not an expert on this topic. I am not even an expert on how to write a curriculum. But let me tell you some other things about myself, and other topics, which have helped me in putting this thing together.

I can speak from experience. I attended the St. Mary's Roman Catholic Indian Residential School from September 1952 to June 1959. In September 1959, I went away to school in Saskatchewan for one year. I came back to St. Mary's in September of 1960. I finally finished my grade 12 in 1964 at St. Mary's.

Some of my classmates were Joe Crop Eared Wolf Jr., Urban Calling Last, Peter Weasel Head, Bruno Many Bears, Andy Crop Eared Wolf, Mary "Lulu" Heavy Shields, Dorothy Rabbit, Doreen (Many Fingers) Rabbit, Louise (Wolf Child) Day Rider, and John Many Chief Jr. I am one of the faces in a framed graduation picture which hung for the longest time at the high school here.

My time at residential school was a jumble of experiences. There were good and bad times, and there were good and bad people. My definition of "bad" people were people who thwarted your happiness. These kinds of people did not want you to feel good about yourself. They just wanted to put down and humiliate you. They could not put you down enough.

The effect that this had on myself and my contemporaries was long-lasting. In spite of the presence of positive people and positive experiences, it seemed that these were not great enough to overcome the negative. The effect was long-lasting and destructive. To this day there are times when I have to convince myself that I am a worthwhile individual, that I am a good person.

I am a Kainaikoan who was born at the Blood Indian Hospital on August 23, 1944. From the day I was born until I went to school in September 1952, I lived at home with my parents and my siblings. Home was a three-room wooden house, which already had a history by the time I was born.

Naahsiksi Morris and Anne Many Fingers built the house and lived in it for some time before they gave it to my parents. My parents got married on Christmas Day, 1934. They lived in the circle of my mother's family for a while before they lived apart from them. When they did, home was a part of the "dowry" my grandfather gave to my mother, along with horses and cattle.

It was to this place that my parents brought me after my mother and I were released from the hospital, probably in September 1944. Although no one lives there anymore, the house still stands today. It is located about four kilometres southwest of where Kainai High School stands today. In my childhood it was located two miles southwest of St. Mary's Roman Catholic Indian Residential School. It stands in the same place.

The house sits on a slight rise, just before the land begins to dip into the valley of the Bull Horn. When all I spoke was Blackfoot, we called it the Pomiipisskaan. Pomiipisskaan is the name of the creek. As you drive by the Senator Gladstone Hall today, there is a sign which says, "Layton Creek." Since our name for this creek predates the white settlement of southern Alberta, "Pomiipisskaan Creek" should be on that sign instead of "Layton Creek." It must have been a fairly old creek already then because it had its own valley where it twisted like Father Lacombe's catechism serpent.

Some of the land features which were important to me as a child were Pomiipisskaan to the east, tatsikihkimiko, a'kiito, paaksipa to the south, and poksikaawahko and omahksikaawahko to the west. For some reason, I cannot recall anything memorable located to the north. However, in the distance I could see Mookoansiistsi, the Belly Buttes.

When I was a child I referred to Pomiipisskani, tatsikihkimikoyi, a'kiitoyi and paaksipay without considering anything else about them, such as what they meant. It was only way later, when I was much into adulthood, that I found out that Pomiipisskaan meant something like "fatty/greasy buffalo jump," tatsikihkimikoi meant "hill at center of flat," a'kiitoi was "wooded area on the side of a hill," and paaksipaa is hickory or a similar type of tree.

I doubt that the really big tree which grew here was a hickory tree but it was huge and it grew out from the side of a hill. Eventually, over a period of many years, it finally toppled into a bend of the Pomiipisskaan. In doing so, it formed a natural bridge which was never readily accessible from the west because there was such a thick growth of siinikskaahko on the west side of the creek. To get to it easily, you had to be on horseback.

We used to refer to the omahksikaawahko and poksikaawahko to the west of our home when we talked in terms of distance from the house. For example, if we said that the horses were closer to the poksikaawahko, that meant they were close to the house. And if we said they were closer to the omahksikaawahko, this meant they were farther away.

Before I was eight years old there were only a few times I was away from my home. Three of these times were when my brothers Bernard, Roy and Arnold were each born. My dad took us to our grandparents' place (Many Fingers) when my mother was due to give birth. A fourth time was when I was four or five years old and I ended up in the hospital for about ten days.

My dad and my uncle John had herded some horses into our corral by the barn. Neither of them saw me as I left the house and approached the corral from the south. By the time that they did see me, I was in the path of the herd of horses as they were jumping and running free after they were released from the corral. A particularly mean stallion took exception to my presence and kicked me on the head. I must have been leaning over to my right side with my head bent down when this happened because the scar on the top of my head is a little to the left.

I don't have any recollection of the accident except that I have a memory in my mind of a small boy who is standing in the way of stampeding horses while male voices are yelling at him to get out of the way! When I came out of my coma four or five days later, I don't know what I said or did. However, I do remember, sometime later, my dad holding me up and my mother standing a few feet away urging me to walk to her. When I did, I fell! My right leg was much shorter than my left one.

It was only later that I understood why one leg was shorter. It had something to do with trauma and nerves. I don't know how soon it was that my grandfather began to drive me to Lethbridge every week to see Dr. Mervin, who was a chiropractor. Nitsitaotoipiksskino'tooko ("I went to have my vertabrae adjusted").

After stripping buck-naked, I would be placed on a special table. The doctor would adjust me here and there, all the time telling me to relax. In the end, I would be placed on my stomach and he would exert much pressure around where my back ends and my buttocks begin. This sudden pressure caught me off guard at the beginning, but not so later on. There was always a crackling sound when he did this and something inside me was adjusted.

This was sometimes a painful experience and quite a few times I came out of the doctor's office with tears in my eyes. Unfortunately for me, Dr. Mervin died before my treatment was completed. The result was that my right leg was still about an inch shorter than my left leg. But my limp was not as bad as before. Even to this day, someone who is not familiar with me will ask why I am limping, believing that the cause was only recent and temporary.

This limp was later to become a source of embarrassment when a thoughtless student would imitate my limp to get a laugh from others. As much as a tried, I always felt as if this was my fault. It is only now, when I am much older and I have accepted my other imperfections, that this does not bother me anymore.

For the rest of these eight years I was happy and carefree. I did not go to school earlier than when I did because of the accident. My parents wanted me to be as well as possible. They were also cautious because the doctor who treated me after the horse accident told my parents that I might be slow or unable to learn (because of the destruction of body cells caused by the kick).

Prior to my going to school, my life was simple and uncomplicated. When I woke up in the morning I knew what my day was going to be like.

I knew that whatever happened I would be safe. I would enjoy the food that my mother cooked. I would do chores that my father assigned me to do. One of these was milking the big cow with the pink, chappy teats. I didn't care for this too much as sometimes I must have pinched the cow because it would kick back and cause the milk pail to spill. But I still enjoyed each day that I lived at home.

During my last free summer, which was the summer of 1952, my older brothers Norbert and Tony warned me about school. "Those nuns are terrible, they're mean!" one said. "The food is awful! You won't like it but you'll be forced to eat it!" In my naiveté, I could not fathom food tasting bad because everything that I had ever eaten tasted good to me.

About the nuns I didn't know what to think.

I don't want to make my life seem so insulated before I went to school, but it must have been. The only other time I had ever encountered a white woman, outside of the nuns at the hospital, was on one of the chiropractor trips to Lethbridge. This encounter took place when I accidentally bumped into this naapiaakii in a department store.

I had been walking slowly down the aisles between counters, which held hundreds of shiny and colourful objects. I was so engrossed in my wonder that I did not see this woman until I felt a push and I looked up. Her right arm was raised as if she was going to hit me! I just continued to look at her. She eventually did not hit me.

When I was child both of my parents worked very hard. They had sheep, pigs, chickens, horses and cattle. They grew carrots and potatoes. My dad also farmed some of his land. We were not rich in any sense of the word, but my parents worked hard. Mother always said that if my dad had not been so generous he probably would have accumulated wealth.

However that was not the case. But we did not lack food. Even though we only had a three-roomed house, and we had no electricity and no indoor plumbing, our house was a happy home. (Years later when I lived there for a while, the good spirit of the house was still there. It still contained the warmth established by my grandparents and later by my parents and my brothers and sisters).

My birthday is in the latter part of August. Every year on that day, to celebrate my birthday, my dad would take all of us to Aakaohkiimiiiksi (Cardston) to see a movie. After watching the movie I was given some money to buy whatever junk food I wanted. My mother would also bake a cake for me that day.

On one of my birthdays as we were driving through pastures sodden with recent heavy rain. My dad said something like, "Iitaomainawa'so'p ai'ksistsikomio'ki." He was referring to the fact that if it had been another day, we would probably just have stayed at home. Because it was my birthday, however, we were driving on the wild prairie grass, meandering around little gumbo ponds. The roads, which were actually trails, had soaked up too much water and were too sticky to drive on. Or, they were underwater. This special effort he was making was because it was my birthday, and I wanted to go to a show in Cardston!

Somehow, this memory has always remained in my mind. It might have been my eighth birthday, the last birthday I had before I lost my freedom. Whenever I think about it, I can remember us in our old Chevrolet pickup. My parents, my siblings and myself were driving to Aakaohkiimiiksi. The sound of the soggy earth as it was run over by the rubber tires was unique to itself. This was coupled with the drone of the truck engine. Our little truck must have looked like an ant or some other insect to a spirit in the sky as it moved this way and that way, obviously with a destination in mind.

Shortly after this day, our family made another trip. This one was to Lethbridge to shop for our school clothes. Among the purchases my parents made for me was a pair of Wrangler jeans and a new blue and white shirt with a sky and cloud design on it. Then I had a pair of oxfords, socks, T-shirt and undershorts. My brothers and I each also got an overall jacket. On a later day but soon after, we made the trip to the residential school.

I don't know if it was a Sunday that our parents brought us to St. Mary's. For my older brothers it was to return to school. For me, it was to start school. I remember Father LaFrance meeting us at the top of the front steps. He was the principal, the school administrator, and it seemed everything else. "Hello George," he was saying to my dad as we ascended the steps. My brothers and I were mostly quiet.

It seemed like the process of dropping us off was a fairly short one. In no time the supervisor nun of the small boys had me in a storeroom. From the shelves of clothing in there, she selected a shirt, pants, underwear, socks and shoes. Then she took me to the playroom where I undressed and removed all of my own clothes. I put on my "everyday clothes."

After I got the clothes, each item was marked with indelible black ink and my number was printed on each. My number was "51." This later became indelibly imprinted in my mind, as I had to respond to it whenever our clothes were washed and handed out. "Number 51!" the supervisor yelled out on these occasions. After the first or second time, I responded automatically. From that first time when I went to St. Mary's as a student, my life changed radically. For ten months of the year I no longer lived at home. For ten months of the year I lived my life according to the whims of an institution.

A brass handbell woke us up each morning at 6:00. We had to get up immediately, make up our bed and get into line to wash up. Within sixty minutes all of us were washed, dressed and lined up to go to chapel for mass. After mass we went to the refectory to eat a strange breakfast. For the first time in my life I tasted bad food!

Then we went back to our playrooms to do our chores. Some had to sweep the stairs. Others had to sweep the hallways. More had to clean the playroom and the washroom. By the time these were completed, school was ready to begin. Then we lined up again and marched two-by-two to the H-Block where all the classrooms were then located.

Because both of my grandmothers were half-breed, or because that mad horse kicked my brains right, I did not have too much of a problem learning English. Prior to the time I went to school, I knew only Blackfoot. That was the only language which our parents spoke to us at home. That was the language of our grandmothers and our grandfathers.

I did not mind that part of my school life. Contrary to what the doctor feared after my horse accident, I was able to learn. Because of this, most of my teachers treated me fairly well. Throughout my school life there I even skipped a couple of grades. In one of these, I missed Mr. Cody's grade four class. From what I had heard from the other students, about how he hit and harassed students, I considered myself very lucky.

In any event, I am a "residential school survivor" and, as I have previously stated, some of the long-term effects of the experience are still with me. But they are not overpowering anymore. I thank Ihtsipaitapiiyio'pa for giving me the strength to overcome these. I am also thankful for being born in a community where there are people who help. I refer especially to the elders.

The fact that our language and culture are still alive reassures me. Having these enables me to look at life differently. I am better able to understand more of it. It also gives me a sense of peace and a sense that life is eternal.

Whenever I see a young Niitsitapi person, I wonder what thoughts are inside her or his mind. Many times I see happiness in the eyes. Many times I think I see questions. Sometimes I see a sadness or something troubling. I wonder what has caused this.

To young Niitsitapi, I hope that you will be given some insight as you go through this curriculum with your teacher. I hope that it will cause you to think about different things. You live in a time that is very different from the era of the Indian residential school. But it is important for you to know that what happened in the past has had some effect on the present.

Our people have gone through a lot of negative experiences, and we are still going through a lot. Yet we survive. What is it which keeps us going?

About the Program

Kipaitapiiwahsinnooni is a Blackfoot word which means "our life, our way of life." It refers to the Niitsitapi traditional way of life, which includes the Blackfoot language and culture. It is an inclusive term used by speakers of the language to indicate a common bond. Kipaitapiiwahsinnooni is the title of this curriculum.

Kipaitapiiwahsinnooni is an alcohol and drug abuse education curriculum aimed to assist the young Niitsitapi person to make positive choices about life. By knowing more about his people's spirituality and his people's history, this person will be able to cope with Niitsitapi society and the larger society beyond the borders of the reserve.

Kipaitapiiwahsinnooni will also help students understand themselves and seriously consider the process they are going through as they prepare themselves for the future. This curriculum will help to empower students because they will identify with the society they will inherit. They will understand the nature of change and their relationship to it. They will also understand that they can play positive roles in this change process.

Kipaitapiiwahsinnooni will arm students with knowledge, which they will be able to use later on as adults.

Kipaitapiiwahsinnooni is geared for Niitsitapi students in high school. It may be adapted for non-Niitsitapi students. It may also be used in other areas of the total school curricula as determined by the teacher.

This curriculum is being developed to address some of the inter-generational effects of the boarding school era. Loss of language and culture, and spiritual and cultural shame are some of these effects. Their presence contributes to a lack of a positive personal identity.

The knowledge of Niitsitapi was utilized to create the bulk of this curriculum. Very little was gathered from published sources. Since this curriculum is being developed to help young Niitsitapi, it only made sense.

The lessons utilize activities. Lessons are also planned so that students become involved in evaluating their own learning experiences.

In the past, elders and parents talked to the youth constantly and expected that their advice would be heeded. Regrettably, this practice has largely been discarded over the past two generations. Maybe this curriculum will make up for some of this loss.

History of Residential Schools on Kainaissksaahkoyi

Alcohol and drug abuse have been cited as a coping strategy for many of the ills which plague First Nation reserves in Canada. One of the causes for this abuse is the legacy of Indian residential schools. On Kainaissksaahkoyi there were two such institutions.

The federal government, in conjunction with the Anglican and Roman Catholic churches, operated two residential schools on the Blood Reserve—St. Paul's Anglican Indian Residential School and the St. Mary's Roman Catholic Indian Residential School. At their inception, these schools were set up as mission schools. St. Paul's became a residential school in 1893. It was located at Omahksini ("Big Island," located west of Aakaiksamaiksi or what is today known as the Old Agency area of the reserve). St. Mary's began as the Immaculate Conception School. It opened as a residential school in 1898 and was located in what is now referred to as Lower Standoff, west of the Trading Post.

The heyday of the Indian residential schools on the Blood Reserve began in the 1920s when both schools were relocated closer to the town of Cardston. They were moved away from the influence of the town of Fort Macleod, on the north side of the reserve, to that of the town of Cardston which is located on the south side of the reserve. This move was motivated by politics. The federal government had wanted to sell a large portion of the northeast section of the Blood Reserve. The new St. Paul's Anglican Indian Residential School was completed in 1924. The new Roman Catholic school, renamed as St. Mary's Roman Catholic Indian Residential School, was completed in 1926.

Students who experienced the move to the new schools were amazed at the difference between the old and the new sites. A former student of St. Paul's said that she felt like she had gone to heaven when she arrived at the new school because the building was warm—there was electricity and indoor plumbing. Many students were fascinated by the indoor bathrooms! While there was an improvement in the physical facilities of these residential schools, other aspects of these schools were not so pleasant. Many of the students suffered traumas which would stay with them for a lifetime. Their children were also affected by how they coped with the aftermath of the residential school. In many cases, former students turned to alcohol so that they could forget the shame and suffering they had endured while in residential school. They turned to alcohol to cover the resentment, anger, helplessness and betrayal that they had gone through.

They also turned to alcohol because the residential schools had not sufficiently prepared them for the new society. Most students were trained only to do manual labour. These schools had only succeeded in creating an overwhelming sense of low self-esteem in many students. Some would die from this. Others survived but were miserable in their survival. Some would somehow find a way out of their misery.

Surprisingly, there are some students who remember mostly positive experiences. For a number of reasons, these students may not have suffered as much as others did. The presence of older siblings may have saved them from bullies. Their parents may have been outspoken people who refused to be dominated by anyone, including the school administration. Because parents may have been early and strong adherents of the denomination of the school, the principal and staff of the school may have felt compelled to protect their children (one survivor referred to these people as "church goers"). Whatever the reason, these students also had luck on their side.

By the late 1950s, the federal government's Indian policy had changed from one of isolation to one of integration. This had an effect on the two schools on the Blood Reserve. St. Paul's Indian Residential School was discontinued as a school in 1957. Almost without a whimper, it seemed, it was dead as a residential school. It became a hostel for some students who went to school in Cardston.

St. Mary's was a different story. Due to the strong lobby of the Oblate Fathers in Ottawa, along with the federal Department of Indian Affairs and the support of parents of students attending St. Mary's, the school continued. The latter had been more motivated by the spectre of a community with no high school than by the loss of a Catholic residential school.

These parents were not willing to lose their school and be forced to send their children to outside schools. In any event, by the late 1960s, the school had undergone a change. Chief among its new features was that it was no longer a residential school in the old sense. The residence became a student hostel. It was there mainly for the convenience of students whose homes were too far away from the school. It was also there for students who needed a home of sorts.

Part of this curriculum includes the interviews of former residential school students. The interviews are from former students of both residential schools on the Blood Reserve. These interviews include the varied perception of former students—those who suffered and those who enjoyed the experience.

About the Writer

Leo Fox (Makai'stoo), the writer of the Kipaitapiiwahsinnooni Alcohol and Drug Abuse Education Program was born on August 23, 1944. He is a member of the Blood Tribe and has resided for most of his life on the Blood Reserve. His mother, Piiaakii (Margaret Many Fingers Fox) was from the Mamioyiiksi (Fish Eaters) clan and his father, George Fox was from the Aakaipokaiksi (Many Children) clan.

In December, 1999 he was seconded to the Kainai Board of Education office to write this curriculum. For the previous seventeen years, he had been the principal of the Aahsaopi (Levern) Elementary School in Issoitapi on the Blood Reserve. He enjoyed the years he spent there. He became acquainted with the parents and the students of Aahsaopi who came from all parts of Kainaissksaahkoyi.

For most of his student days, he attended the St. Mary's Roman Catholic Indian Residential School on the Blood Reserve.

About the Artist

Allen Wells was born on March 4, 1957. His mother is from the Blackfeet Reservation in Montana and his father is from the Blood Reserve. He attended the St. Mary's High School on the Blood Reserve and the F.P. Walshe School in Fort Macleod.

He has had no formal art education/training. He is a self-taught artist. "It was always in me to draw. In school that's all I did. In grade 10 I realized what I wanted was to be an artist and I have never looked back," he says.

Allen has experimented with a lot of mediums. His rock art has taken him to places like the Pendleton Roundup in Oregon; the National and the International at Spruce Meadows; and the World All-Indian Rodeo Finals in Saskatoon, Reno and Rapid City to name a few. He has had his art published in *The Western Horseman*. He represented the Blood Tribe at the Calgary Stampede in 1977. More recently, his logo submission to the 2002 World Indigenous Peoples' Conference on Education was chosen as the official one.

Allen says, "I am proud to be part of this book. I think it will help our people regain their identity now and in the future. I have a son named A.J. and I am very proud of him. I thank all the people who have supported me through the years. Thank you especially to the good Lord."

Allen also had a daughter named Charmayne who was killed in an auto accident when she was two years of age.

GOAL(S)

Students will understand how Niitsitapiaatsimoihkaani (our way of prayer) is based on nature.

OBJECTIVE(S)

1. Students will discuss why Nato'si (the sun) is an important part of our prayers.
2. Students will explain why respect for nature is part of our prayers.
3. Students will tell how healers received their power to heal.
4. Students will explain why we ask our departed relatives to help us in our prayers.
5. Students will determine how Niitsitapiaatsimoihkaani is inclusive.
6. Students will compose a personal prayer incorporating the elements of nature and respect.

CULTURAL CONCEPT

Niitsitapiaatsimoihkaani is our way of prayer. It is natural and it is based on respect for nature.

STUDENT ACTIVITIES

1. Students will listen to the cultural background information as their teacher reads it.
2. Students will have a short class discussion.
3. In cooperative groups of four, students will design a poster depicting Niitsitapiaatsimoihkaani.
4. When the posters are completed students will explain their posters.
5. Students will research the river systems in Alberta, for example, where they begin and where the tribes of Niitsitapi are located. This will be a comprehensive project which will look at dams, livestock production, location of towns and cities, etc.

EVALUATION ACTIVITIES

1. Students will be graded on the research project. Evaluation will be based on how comprehensive the project is.
2. Students will work in their cooperative groups to design a test. They will give this test to all other students.

RESOURCES

1. Elders from Iitskinayiiksi and Mao'to'kiiksii and bundle holders

NIITSITAPIAATSIMOIHKAANI (OUR WAY OF PRAYER)

CULTURAL BACKGROUND INFORMATION

It is what we were given. We were placed here with it. There is nothing complex about it.

When we pray we call on the sun "Ayo, ayo naapi Naato'si…" The reason we do this is because the sun gives us day, it gives us light, it brings light to everything. It is what the one who was here and who went back into the heavens gave us. It is the source of life that we depend on.

We learn about life and understand our place in it because we call on Naapi Naato'si. We call on the sun for help and to the holy ones Ksaahkommiitapiiwa.

Without the sun, there would only be darkness. It would be very bleak. In the evening, kipitaakii Ko'komiki'somm takes over and provides light at night. She guides the night and allows the dream spirits to come to us in our sleep.

Our way of prayer teaches us to respect everything. The reason for this is because everything that exists has a reason for being.

When the Creator placed us here, he did the same thing with the land animals, the flying animals and the animals that live in the water. Also, the rivers and mountains and everything else were put here. That is why we value these things. That is why we must look after them.

The water that we drink, the water that flows down the mountains, gives sustenance to the plants and trees. These plants and trees provide some of the food which we and the animals eat. Some of the animals provide the meat that we eat.

People slept in isolated locations looking for spirit helpers. Different animals gave their gifts and became spirit helpers to some who sought this. This is where the healers got their ability to heal the sick and the injured.

The ones who have left us and gone before us return to goodness. They join and become members of the holy ones. "Listen to us, we call on you for help," we say to them.

We all pray to the same power, to the one who plans all things. We have our ceremonies in how we honour the one who controls all things. Others have their own ways. But we all pray to the Creator.

It is not good to argue about prayer, however way it is offered. We should unite in ensuring that we all value prayer. Then we will be all related with each other.

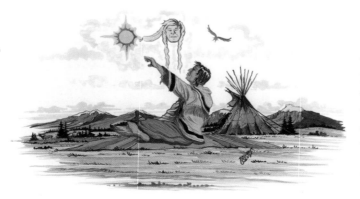

The people prayed to Ihtsipaitapiiyiopa and to Naato'si. In their prayers they included the water, the mountains and the earth. All the birds and land animals were also mentioned. Paramount in our prayers was the search for harmony in our relationships with others.

GOAL(S)

1. To understand Niitsitapi spirituality.
2. To understand how animals influenced Niitsitapi spirituality.
3. To understand the concepts of honesty and faithfulness.

OBJECTIVE(S)

1. Students will know the story of how the O'kaan started.
2. Students will know the requirement for performing the O'kaan.
3. Students will develop respect for each other.

CULTURAL CONCEPT

Our sacred ceremonies were received from the animal world. The elk gave us the O'kaan ceremony.

STUDENT ACTIVITIES

1. The students will listen to the story of how O'kaan was gifted to Niitsitapi.
2. Rosie Day Rider or another elder will talk to the students about the O'kaan.
3. Students will discuss the story.
4. In cooperative groups of four, students will illustrate the story with captions.

EVALUATION ACTIVITIES

1. Students will correctly answer a short quiz on the O'kaan story including details about the name of the ceremony, the animal who gave us the ceremony, the circumstances of the story and the outcome.
2. Students will write a short reflective paper beginning with "The O'kaan story taught me that..."

RESOURCES

1. Kainai elders: Rosie Day Rider, Margaret Hind Man, Bruce Wolf Child, recorded interview with Rosie Day Rider

HOW THE O'KAAN WAS GIVEN TO NIITSITAPI

CULTURAL BACKGROUND INFORMATION

In the O'kaan (Chaste Woman Ceremony), a woman who can profess that she knows only her husband in the sexual way can do this ceremony. Like other ceremonies which our people have, this one to came from the animal world.

The animal involved in the O'kaan was the elk.

In a herd of elk in the mountains was a family made up of a male elk, his female partner and their offspring, a young male elk. The older elk was not totally secure about his relationship with his wife. As time went by he felt unsure about his partner's love and devotion. Consequently, he led his family away from the herd.

When they had been gone for the period of a moon phase, the young male elk expressed dissatisfaction with their location. "Why are we here away from the others?" he asked his mother one day. She didn't know the reason why but she told her son she would ask his dad. "Why have we been gone from the others so long?" she asked him. "Our son is losing weight because he is unhappy about not being with his relatives and friends."

"You are the one who is missing her male friends. You are using your son as an excuse to return to your boyfriends," he answered her. The female elk was stunned and affronted by his answer. So that was why they had been gone from the rest of the herd for so long! Her woman's intuition had alerted her that something might be bothering her husband. Still, she was insulted.

"I have never fooled around with anyone and I have been faithful to you from the start," she told him. "I have known no other male but yourself. We will have a contest to see who is telling the truth. Whoever is telling the truth will be able to topple that big tree over there."

The male elk looked at the tree she was talking about. It was a large poplar tree which stood away from the others. "Hah," he grunted. "No tree, no matter how big, could withstand the force of his physical strength," he thought.

Because he was so proud and sure of himself, he did not psyche himself up or do any other form of preparation before he attempted to meet the challenge issued by his mate. He charged toward the tree. The pain! The explosion of light on impact! Only his male ego kept him from going down. The impact of his head ramming against the tree had almost taken his antlers off. The poplar tree stood silent and motionless.

The female elk waited while her mate cleared his mind. Then she prepared to take her turn. With super concentration she dug her hooves into the mossy mountainous terrain and slowly walked toward the tree. Four times she positioned herself and made the motions as if to hit the tree. Then she struck! As if in slow motion, the poplar tree lost its grip on the earth and was totally uprooted.

The male elk was chagrined by his wife's strength. But the truth about her character was greater than his feeling of humiliation. "You are telling the truth. We will go back to the others," he told her.

This is how the O'kaan came to be.

RESIDENTIAL SCHOOL INTERVIEW

ELDER/SURVIVOR A

I went to the St. Paul's Anglican Residential School from 1936 to 1945. I was forced to go by Canon Middleton. My father said it was time to go to school. My mother said that if I didn't go to school Dad would go to jail. She said, "If you want Dad to go to jail then don't go to school. Who will look after us? What will happen to us?" There was no other school which I could have attended.

1936–1945

At the school we had reading, numbers, math and how to pray. To this day I can't read very well. I really didn't learn very well. At the school I was in the classroom for half a day. The other half I worked in the kitchen, the laundry, or I did general housekeeping work.

I spoke only Blackfoot when I went to school. At home it was the only language spoken because my dad and grandparents had never gone to school. Mom went to school but she didn't speak to us in English.

When I went to school I could not use Blackfoot anymore. If I did, I was slapped around, made to stand in the corner, scrub floors and write lines on the blackboard. I had to write "I will speak English all day". If the lines began to slant as I got tired, the teacher would erase all that I had written and I would have to begin all over again.

I learned a little English. I could read some and write a little. I also learned some life skills. This was what was good about my school experience. However, there were too many bad things about my school experience. We couldn't play or fool around. We couldn't run, we had to walk. We were never shown any affection. Our mistakes were always spoken about in public. The staff was never satisfied. They cut my hair. They said that we were not allowed to wear braids. I was slapped because I cried when they cut my hair!

I feel real good about our spirituality and our way of praying. I was raised that way. I don't really practice the Anglican religion anymore but I do go there.

I suffered physical and emotional abuse. I will never forget what happened to me. I was not developing physically as the other girls were doing. I did not begin to menstruate when the other girls began theirs. They teased me and gossiped about me. The supervisors, staff, teachers would ask me in front of the whole class if I was pregnant. One time, the supervisor grabbed me between the legs to check to see if I had started my periods. I was even brought to the hospital. The nuns gave me a drink of castor oil so that I would start. This went on for some time. When I did start the teasing from the other students and humiliation by the staff did not stop. The sisters said that I had miscarried and that was why I finally started. I was so scared and lonely.

I saw other students being abused too. One of my friends worked in the bakery. Sometimes, when she finished work, the supervisor would give her some bread with real butter on it. One day I was waiting for her to finish work. I waited in the hallway when she walked out of the kitchen. Another supervisor who was just leaving her room across the hallway saw my friend with the bread. She didn't talk to my friend. She didn't even ask her how she had gotten the bread. She just started to hit her and slap her. She tore the bun apart and shoved the crusty side into my friend's mouth. My friend began to choke and she couldn't breathe. I tried to push the supervisor away but she continued to shove the bread into her mouth. Finally, I was able to get the bread out of her mouth. From that time on my friend was always scared and nervous. She never wanted to be alone. Even at night, we would push our beds together and I would hold her hand through the night. Sometimes I would have to tell her not to cry or make any noises. I wished that my mom or dad would take me out of there.

Because of the way I was treated at the school, I lost all respect for myself. I don't know myself. I can't show love to my kids. I always have a wall between myself and the people I love, as well as my friends. I lost a lot of beliefs about life. I don't know how to share. I lost everything. Love and sharing mean a lot. I was raised by the residential school staff who were supposed to help me. Instead, they caused me to have a hard life today.

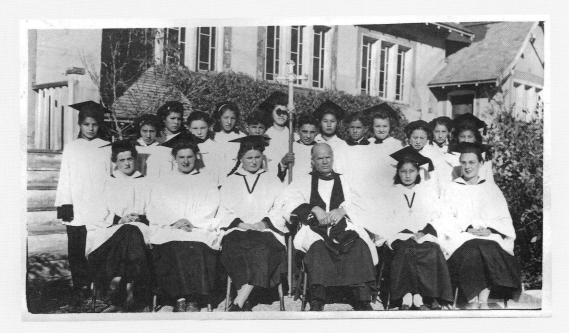

St. Paul's School Choir with S.H. Middleton in front row, circa 1940s.

RESIDENTIAL SCHOOL INTERVIEW

ELDER/SURVIVOR B

I attended the St. Mary's Roman Catholic Indian Residential School from 1946 to 1952. We had no choice, we had to go to school. My parents were Catholic and we were not allowed to go to the white schools. I left school at the age of sixteen. I went up to grade six. The residential school went up to grade eight at the time.

They taught us math, spelling, reading and social studies. They also taught us the Catholic religion (catechism). I was also taught how to sew. I never worked in the kitchen as some girls did, so I never learned how to cook there. My mother taught me how to cook at home.

Other than sewing, the teaching was not really useful for me.

When I went to school I spoke only Blackfoot. It was the only language we spoke at home. We were not allowed to speak our own language in the school. If we did speak it, one of the consequences was that we would have to stand in a corner. Another punishment was that we would have to go without a meal.

When we'd be out in the playground we would talk Blackfoot because no nuns would be around. Also, we'd steal a loaf of bread from the bakery which was on our way as we went out to the playground. The girls who worked in the bakery after school would hand us a loaf of bread through one of the windows. Occasionally we did get caught, but most of the time we didn't. Then we'd have a feast with our bread in the playground. Times like this, being amongst my friends, were some of my happy times.

I used to get very lonely. On Sundays when my parents came to visit us and when they were leaving to go home, I used to run after them. They had a buggy and a team of horses. Sometimes they'd take me home with them but most of the time they'd take me back to school. Another thing that was not good was that the nuns were very strict. We could never talk to or look at the boys. If we did we would get a slap in the face. Also, we never had enough to eat. We were always hungry.

I feel good about our Indian religion. I believe in it. But I also still practice being a Roman Catholic. I still attend church and say the rosary.

1946–1952

I was abused when I was in residential school. I was slapped on the face and I was pushed around. That's what would happen if we got caught talking Blackfoot, talking to or even just looking at the boys. We were not allowed to use the bathroom anytime we needed to go. We could only use it at certain times. The washroom was always locked.

I saw other students being strapped. I also saw others standing in the corner or not having a meal. This could have been any one of the three meals. In the classroom, if we were questioned and we didn't know the answer, we'd get punished. We would probably miss recess, get a good lecture about studying, and we'd have to do lines (write a sentence 100 or 200 times).

My residential school days were one of my best times in spite of all the abuse we suffered. We did a lot of things we were told not to do and we did not get caught. Of course you would have to be with your best friend because you knew she wouldn't tell on you. But, on the other hand, if someone else saw you or heard about something you were not supposed to do or say, there would be lots of trouble.

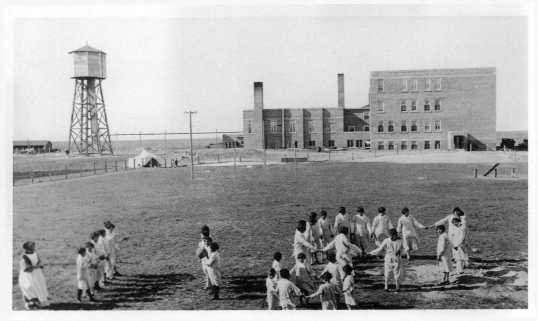

St. Mary's Residential School playground.

RESIDENTIAL SCHOOL INTERVIEW

ELDER/SURVIVOR C

1940

I went to residential school also. I went to school when the war started. The government decided that when an Indian child was seven years old, that child had to start attending school.

There were many of us in my family. Work was not as easily available then as it is now. You people will get up in the morning and you will go to work. It was not like that in the past. The only time there was work was in the spring when crops were being planted and in the fall when crops were being harvested. Haying took place in the summer. Then there were those who did work in the commercial gardens. Work was seasonal.

When we went to school our parents were saved the expense of looking after us. We had it good. We were fed, we had a place to sleep, and the school was very clean.

Our supervisors were very diligent in their work. They talked to us about life and what we needed to know to live a good and clean life. The principal did the same thing, he talked to us.

There were fun activities for us there too. For example, there was a school orchestra and people from outside used to come to listen to us play in concerts at Christmas and Easter. We were taught to play instruments.

Prayer was a big part of my school experience. Prayer is good because it connects us to the Creator. It made us live a good life. Today's children are very different. They have not been taught prayer and their lives are so directionless.

I did not go very far academically. When I was eleven years old I had to go away to a hospital for treatment of an illness I had. I was gone for three years, after which I returned to the school.

School at that time did not only mean book learning. We had to work in the kitchen, in the sewing room and in the laundry. Then there were those who were assigned to do general cleaning of the school. We had to do these different work assignments so that we could be independent later on.

I can honestly say that what I learned at the residential school helped me. I was able to work for many years because of the skills I received in residential school. I have a pension today because of the many years I worked.

I have heard people say that the food we ate at residential school was bad. Yet, when I went there, I never knew anyone who was poisoned by the food we ate. The school menu was always improving. When I began to work there in 1954 the food served to the children was good. I think that there have been some misleading statements made about this.

I remember some of the children who went to school there who have become leaders in our community. They learned useful things when they went to school. It was not all bad. I cannot say that my residential school experience was bad.

Of course there were the bullies. They were the ones who made our lives miserable. They made our lives more miserable than did the nuns and priests. When we were punished there was a reason for this punishment. We learned respect and how to listen to our elders.

I noticed the change in student behavior from the earlier residential school era and the later day-school students. Whereas the former were orderly and respectful, that latter were loud and disrespectful. Very few of the students knew basic manners. I think that the parents who went to residential school were good parents. I think that they raised their children to be respectful.

In our family, our parents raised us to love each other. If we fought with each other we were strapped on the legs. Most of my siblings are still alive and we have arguments. But we don't allow these arguments to turn into feuds. We are still close.

Parenting has really changed today. It seems that many parents do not discipline their children at all. Many children threaten their parents with child abuse charges if there is any chance of corporal punishment being done by parents.

Something has to change. Too many children do not realize the risks that exist today. Because they are allowed to do whatever they want, young people do not seem to realize the dangers that lurk out there.

When we were young, our grandparents, mothers and fathers talked to us. They warned us and talked to us all the time.

Parents who work today put too much importance on their careers and not enough on their children. They neglect their children because of their jobs. They have lost their parenting skills.

When I went to school, Blackfoot was my only language. I don't recall being punished for speaking Blackfoot. It is true that we had rules and if we followed these rules we were okay. But if we chose not to follow the rules, we were punished. One of the punishments was we were sent to bed. We did not want to be sent to bed because we were afraid of being alone in the dormitory.

I don't agree with people who are putting a lot of blame on residential schools as the reason for all of our problems. The loss of parenting skills and the social problems like drinking can be blamed on other things.

We didn't ask to have drinking opened for us. A lot of people really began to drink when this was done. In the old days, those people who drank and who got drunk were well known because there were so few people who drank habitually. Fetal alcohol syndrome did not exist in the past because very few women drank.

Because of a lack of job opportunities, with the result that there is nothing else to do, many people drink.

There were not very many single mothers in the old days. Most girls got married at the same time they left school. In fact, when girls reached the age of thirteen, they were not allowed to go home during the summer holidays. They did not get a chance to fool around and a chance to get pregnant.

Now many students are getting pregnant. One mother indicated to me that the reason she enrolled her daughter elsewhere was because of pregnant girls being allowed to stay in school today. She was afraid that the example of the older girls would unduly influence her daughter to do the same.

You don't see too many pregnant high school girls at other schools off the reserve. In the days of the residential school, there were hardly any students who got pregnant while they were still in school.

Based on my own experience, I don't think residential schools were as bad as some people have made them out to be. I think some people have been influenced because of the cash settlements they believe they will be getting.

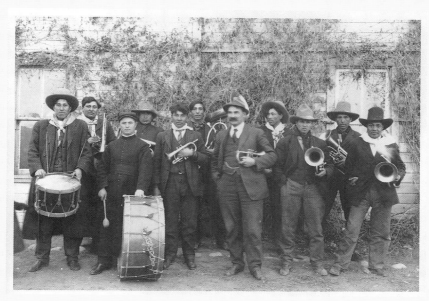

Brass band at Blood Indian Reserve at Cardston.

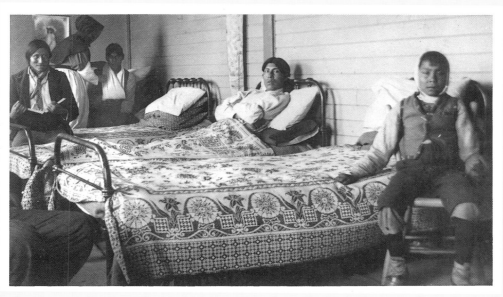

Hospital patients at the Blood Reserve Hospital.

BILL HEAVY RUNNER

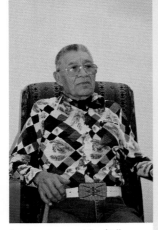

Issokoyioomaahka (Bill Heavy Runner), Kainai elder and grandfather to the Kanattsoomitaiksi.

I have been asked to talk about the traditional way of teaching the young, to enable them to lead a good and orderly life. Old man Issokoyioomahka and Aapiksisskstaki raised me. Both my older sister and I were well raised by these old people.

We were taught everything that they could teach us. I am seventy-nine years old now and I have never been to jail. I have never participated in fighting, stealing, making fun of other people or taking things which did not belong to me. These are Niitsitapissksinima'tstohksini.

I know a lot of the people who were taught in this way. Most of them are gone now. They were good people because of the way they were shown how to live. Many of these people were older than I was. There were some who lived exemplary lives.

A boy was strictly trained. I was taught to get up early. My old man used to tell me to, "Hang up your clothes and put your shoes together before you go to bed. In case we are attacked during the night, you will be able to get them quickly." I was taught as if it was in the warring days, when we fought our enemies incessantly. I guess in those days there were frequent night attacks. A warrior needed to have what he needed close by.

I was taught everything including prayer, Niitsitapiaatsimoihkaani. We were raised with it. I grew up with it.

Early in the morning I had to round up the horses and bring them in. They were our only means of transportation. Life was not that easy. Sometimes in frustration I cried because some of the horses would stray or the air was too cold.

Whenever I was doing something or making something, I was told to be mindful to finish the task. Whenever I used a tool, my grandfather would tell me, "When you have finished using that tool, put it back to where it was before. You will have need for it again in the future. Look after what you use. If you do, you will be able to use it for a long time." If I came across a nail somewhere, my grandfather would tell me to pick it up and save it. I would have need for it sometime in the future.

In the mornings was when my grandfather would talk to me about life. He taught me lessons. He would ask me what my plans were for a day. I would tell him. Then he would say, "There are two ways you can do something. One way is you can do something quickly and finish it quickly. But it will not last. The second way is to do it more carefully. It will become a challenging task. What you are making will last a long, long time because you have made it as well as you can. That is why you have to consider things first. You should not act hastily. Life is like that too. That is why I talk to you all the time."

If we build a house quickly we will notice soon after we move in that there are a lot of things wrong with it. It will not be as warm as we wanted it. Other things will be wrong with it too. Life is like that. Just as if you took the time to build a house carefully and well, so it is life. This is the type of teaching myself and older people were brought up with.

We were brought up with it. "Do not fight with each other. Whenever there is another child around, play with that person. Do not pick on that other child." We grew up with this advice.

As I got a little older, he also talked to me about horses. "Horses are important to us," he told me. When someone does not have a horse, they have a hard time getting around. They are poor. Look after your horses. Treat them right and look after them properly. You will find them useful." I learned to look after my horses properly. In the summer we put up hay because our horses would need it in the wintertime. When someone did not do this, his horses lost weight over the winter and they became very thin.

Whenever I came back from a trip somewhere with my horse, my grandfather told me, "Feed and water your horse before you think about eating." I was mindful of this advice. In the morning, before I ate breakfast, I watered and fed my horse which was tethered. I looked after my horse because I realized it was my only means of transportation.

A properly cared for horse could endure a lot. It could be counted on in an emergency. It would be able to go a long distance if necessary and not tire easily because it was well cared for.

The advice of my grandfather followed me to school when I finally went to school at thirteen years of age. "Do not fight with the other students," he told me. "Learn to read and write as you are supposed to do. You will need these skills in the future. Our way of life is changing, you will need these new skills."

I listened to the advice of my grandfather. The values that he taught me have stood me well over my lifetime. The education he taught me was very high-quality education.

"I have raised you as my children," he told my sister and me. "I talk to you and give you advice because I love you. I want you to have a good life," he said to us. "When we are no longer around, your grandmother and I, you will know what to do. You will not have to look around wondering how to live your life because we have shown you the way," he told us.

All of the people raised their children in this way. They advised them constantly.

When I reached adulthood, I did some crazy things. We all do these things. But I did not steal or fight. I looked after my horses and they were useful to me when I needed them to pull the cultivator, to break up my land and raise grain on it. I was never idle. I always had something to do.

The same can be said of my older sister. Our grandparents advised her constantly as well. My grandmother showed her household skills like washing clothes and sewing. She was also shown how to prepare hides and how to do beadwork. When she was older, she was kept busy because of custom orders people made for her beadwork. She earned some money from it. She learned her other homemaker skills as well.

We were also taught to respect prayer. Whenever someone was praying, we were told to maintain a silence in respect for the ongoing prayer.

If I was going somewhere, my grandfather instructed me to take a warm jacket, "in case of a rainstorm," he would say. On one occasion I did not follow his advice and did not take a jacket with me. On the way home after visiting my friend, a rainstorm overtook me and I was soaked to the bone.

My mother and father did not raise me. It was my grandparents who raised me. By the time of their death, they had given me a lot. I learned so much from their wisdom.

They prayed everyday—in the morning, at noon and in the evening. They smudged their faces with ochre. My grandfather told me, "Naapiikoaiksi pray with the blood of the Creator. We were given the red ochre to use in our prayers." Poisskinaksini or face-painting is still done today. Whenever someone has had a disturbing dream, he/she will ask an omahkitapi to paint their face to ward off any evil which may be lurking around. Aamato'simaani is also used in this ceremony. "Nothing bad will happen to you. Do not worry anymore," the elder says afterward. There were many people who lived well into old age in those days.

My grandparents also advised me to give something to an old person whenever I met one. A small amount of cash or tobacco was a useful gift to an elder. Whenever I gave a gift to an elder, he was always thankful and he prayed for me. "Ayo Spomitapi aamo saahkomaapiw nitsiini'stotook. Kiistoi kimiiksistsini'stotook. Aook ahkihkohtaihtawa'psi mo saahkomaapiw. (Holy Spirits this boy has been kind to me. In reality he is honouring you. Give this boy good luck and long life for giving me this gift)," he prayed. I was also instructed to help them out in other ways whenever I could.

These people showed us how to live life. We survived and lived because of this advice.

We were shown also how to observe the sun's cycle to determine the right time for opening sacred bundles. The elders used sticks called ka'kstaksin on which they marked when the last opening was. The bundles were opened and the contents prayed with each year. They contained the skins and feathers of many different animals and birds. They included ksisskstaki, aimmoniisi, piinotoyi, a'sinnotoyi, sa'aiksi, ayi'sipisaiksi, siikamm, kiitoki, mi'ksikatsi and miisa'ai.

Berry soup was made for the occasion and there was prayer. Each animal within the bundle had a song and, when a song was sung, the owner would identify to which animal the song belonged.

The owner prayed outside when the sun came up. He prayed for everything. His prayers were comprehensive. In his prayers he prayed for the berries, that there were some. This was the ceremonial food. He prayed for the trees. He prayed for the water plants. He prayed that the water which flowed would remain pure enough to drink as long as it flowed in the rivers. He prayed that he would long see the mountains.

We do not exist in isolation from the other living things. My grandfather told me this. He said, "We do not exist by ourselves without the help of other things. This tree here helps us to keep warm because we burn its branches and we use them to make stakes for our tipis to hold them down. The rocks we use to hold things down and to heat our sweat lodges.

The Indian medicines we used we had to dig up. We were taught about them and we dug for them. The old man's medicines were different from the old woman's. My grandfather would say that he was given these plants to use. It was in the fall when we dug for the roots. They grew in particular places, not just anywhere. One type of root which grew in a rocky location, particularly where we hauled water from, was called aiksikkooki. It had a bitter taste. Another root was called sooyiaihts. It was good for burns. We would also spend much time collecting ka'kitsimoi. Ka'ksimiistsi was another plant we harvested. We used it to make a tea in the wintertime especially to help with colds.

All of these things we were told about so that we would be able to make use of them. These helped us with life. We were also taught about the weather so that we knew when there was going to be a storm and when it was going to be cold. Our old people made sure that we had a lot of firewood gathered before winter, so that we wouldn't have to do that after the snow came.

These were the teachings of my old people. They are buried not too far from here. I sometimes go to where they are buried and I talk to them. I thank them for having raised me with such knowledge so that I lived my life properly. "I thank you for the life you gave me. I thank you for showing me the way even after you were gone. I am still living now. I thank you for that"—this is what I say.

I also received ceremonial knowledge. When I was younger I went through a lot of our ceremonies. Now I am able to assist the younger generation as an advisor. When the Kanattsoomitaiksi started up again, there was nobody else around who knew about the society. They called on me to advise them. I am glad I had the knowledge to help them.

Now they meet once a month. I am their advisor. I have helped with face painting. Sometimes Iitskinayiiksi will be undecided about something. They will ask me. When I was younger I was an associate of the Piinotoyi. I danced the circle with the Piinotoyi.

I was instructed about tolerance for others in how they prayed. "Whenever a person is praying," I was told, "do not make fun of them." When I went to school my grandmother told me to listen to the ones known as naatowa'paakiiksi. She told me this because they were our teachers. My grandfather gave me the same advice for naatoyiaapiikoaiksi.

When I went to school we had a priest known as Aahsaopi. This priest knew how to speak Blackfoot and he taught us religion. In his classes he mentioned maka'pato'si (the devil). Sometime later, when I was home, I happened to mention that maka'pato'si was here. My grandfather asked me where I had heard about maka'pato'si. I told him. "Never mention his name in this house again!" he told me. "We have no such person in our way. He is the bad spirit of the naapiikoaiksi," he told me. "They brought him over when they came here."

Later still, I mentioned omahkaohpakoyittsi. My grandfather said, "I want you to learn about good things. That is why I sent you to school. I didn't send you there to learn about bad things. I am going to go to the school to have a talk with them about this. They're the ones who must go to Omahkaohpakoyittsi! Don't mention that place around here."

He later went to the school and told Father Levern not to talk about hell and the devil to the children. He told Father Levern to talk to the children about positive things, not bad things if he wanted them to pray in the white people's way.

We were also raised with sharing and hospitality. When a visitor came even for just a short time he was told, "Sit here. Have some tea." If the person was in a hurry, he would say "Just give me some tea. I am in a hurry." He would mention this act of hospitality later on as he travelled. If he was just visiting he was told, "Sit down. Have something to eat before you leave again." The visitor would be grateful for the hospitality and he would mention that he was fed there.

I still practice this today. "Have some tea," I tell a visitor. If he is in hurry he will tell me. If he doesn't say anything, I will offer him something to eat.

It is a bad practice to ask as visitor, "Would you like something to eat?" This was practised by selfish people in the past. It was a taunt used by aiksimmotsiiksi.

Visitors were also given something. Cloth, for example, was sometimes given. Today I still practice this. Especially when my relatives from Piikani come to visit, I give them money to help them with hotel expenses.

I have three children of my own today. I lost a fourth whom I still regret losing today. Now I have some stepchildren too. When I married their mother, I told them that I would also be their father since their own dad was dead. They respect me.

When someone treats me in a good way, I feel the same way. I feel good. I like to treat others in a good way. My old people used to tell me, "You will not get something from doing bad things. If you carry rumours around, someone will get after you."

When people have gotten after me in the past, I just listened to them without retaliating. I just looked at them. When someone asked for my help, I would help that person. I do not have a lot of money. If I can help someone out with money, I will. Many do not return money I have lent them. I will not go to them and say, "When are you going to return that money I lent you?" When someone returns money, I feel good. The old people used to say, "Money blows by you in the wind. You can always get more."

People helped each other in the past without expecting to get any kind of payment. They just did it. For example, a man helped to cultivate another person's field without expecting anything in return. If there was any kind of payment exchange, it was a bonus for the one helping out.

Help other people without expecting to get paid for it. Feed people who come to your home. These are all things I was instructed to do by my grandparents.

In the days when I was still a dancer, I had a complete outfit. My wife made me a complete dancing outfit. Relatives from the outside visited me and I would give them something from my outfit such as moccasins, headdress or something else. My wife would have to sew a new item to replace the one I had given away.

I did this because of the teaching I got from my grandparents—how to relate to other people, how to understand the weather and to prepare for winter were all things I was taught. I was also told the past-people's stories so that I could understand things better. Included in these stories were the war stories of our people, and what they went through to achieve warrior status.

My grandfather lived on the tail end of those days. He went on his first raid when he was fourteen years old. He and a friend went together. Later on, as they encountered the harsh reality of the trail, they regretted their decision. "Maybe we should have stayed at home," they told each other as their doubts set in.

Men who had had war experiences told their stories. Not only did they relate how they fought, they also told of the misery that they experienced. Then there were the successes they had in war. These were later used to bestow names on younger family members.

For example, one of my names was Niokskaikakato'si (Three Stars). This was a war name. When he went on his first raid, at fourteen years of age, one of the hardships my grandfather experienced was a blizzard. To get out of it, he and his friend built a lean-to. As he was looking out the opening of their temporary shelter he saw a break in the clouds. Inside this break, he saw three stars. On this raid, which was his first, he brought home a pony from an enemy tribe's herd.

When he took my sister and me into his home and decided to raise us, he gave me the name Niokskaikakato'si. A grandfather from Piikani gave me the name Miosskitsipahpi. Another grandfather gave me the name Niistsikapai'pisstsi. Finally, I took another name which is my name now. It is Issokoyioomahka. These were all my names. Now I have given them out to my grandchildren.

I always remember that my grandparents went through hardship to raise me. This is why I have agreed to share this information with you. This was how the old people instructed their young. They always took grandchildren to raise. They had so much compassion. My wife and I have also done this. We more or less adopted a grandson to raise. He was with us until he was older.

Compassion for others was a large component of the training we received from our grandparents. Looking after each other was another part of this training. Being sincere in our responsibility for others was another. This referred in particular to looking after our aged people who are helpless, and to others who cannot really look after themselves.

Prior to my grandfather's death when he was ninety-eight years old, just the two of us lived together. He was not able to do too much for himself then. I looked after him the best way that I could. I remembered all that he had done for me to raise me properly. Now it was my turn to do the same for him. The training he gave me was invaluable. He taught me about everything. His training was very useful for me. I am now sharing it with others.

I was a member of the Kanattsoomitaiksi twice. When I was transferring my membership the second time, my grandfather told me, "Just because you have transferred the rattle of the Kanattsoomitaiksi away now does not mean you have ceased to be a member of that society. People in the future will remember that you were an active member twice. They will come to you for advice in the future.

When I had been a member, I was told that the other members were my like my family. Whenever we met each other we were happy to see each other. We shook hands or we kissed each other. Each time we met, no matter how often, we were glad to see each other.

Today I am a grandfather to the Kanattsoomitaiksi. When they danced last summer at aakokaatsini I noticed how many members there were. They have many members.

I told them that as their adopted grandfather, they were like my children. I am the oldest member. I reminded them to love one another. Whenever they prayed, I told them to pray for simple things, for gentle things. Old man Aapohkiaayo used to tell me the same thing, "Whenever you pray to the Creator, ask for simple things, for gentle things. The Creator looks upon you and he witnesses that you are a kind and gentle person. He will respond to your prayers."

There are some young people who do not know the right way. They do not seem to care if they do or not. There are some parents and grandparents who will not talk to their young people because they do not want to talk to them harshly. If another adult tells them about some wrong that their children have done, they will not listen and ask that nothing be said to the offending children.

This situation can only last for as long as the parents or grandparents are alive. What about when they are gone? Who's going to make excuses for the offending children? What will the children or grandchildren do then?

My grandfather talked to me all the time because he loved me. He cared for me. He was concerned about my future. He used to tell me, "The child who does not listen to his parents or grandparents will get into trouble by himself. The one who listens to his parents or grandparents will have an orderly life."

I think back on some real situations from the past. I recall this one person who came from a very well-to-do family on the reserve. He was an only child. He was not made to work for anything. His father got him whatever he asked for. He asked for a lot. Then the father died. Not too long after that his mother died too. Then there was just himself left alone with all the property. What was he to do? He could not work because his father had only pampered him when he was alive. He did not know what to do. All he could do was to sell the livelihood that his parents had accumulated over their lifetime. He started with the horses and cattle, then the land and the house. In the end he was left with only his body. Kaaksistomiw.

It is important for parents and grandparents to talk to their children all the time. It is also important for children to listen to their parents and grandparents so that they know what to do in the future.

When my grandfather died, he left me with what property he had—horses, cattle, farm implements and so on. When I thought about it, I realized that I had no one to ask for advice. But because he had prepared me well, I relied on the knowledge he had passed on to me and I knew I had to do things on my own now.

There had been one time in my growing up years that I had had "no ears" for my grandfather's advice. I had been at Issoitapi and bet my horse and saddle in a card game. I lost. When I came home on foot, and my grandfather found out what had happened, he was not pleased. When my grandparents found out who won them from me, my grandfather went to get them. He brought another horse as payment for the one I lost.

What had I gained from my gambling? He ridiculed the fact that I had to walk home after I lost my horse and saddle. I had lost an excellent horse and a saddle for nothing! I realized the wisdom of what he was telling me and from that moment on I did not gamble with cards. Every now and then I did play hand games.

The training I got from my grandparents was based on wisdom and truth. My grandfather encouraged me to face hardships and challenges head on. I was never to give up because eventually I would be able to overcome these.

The training I got from my grandfather was comprehensive. I was taught about everything.

I feel a responsibility for my stepchildren. They are also my children now because their natural father is dead. When one of them was going to join the Horn Society, he felt bad because his father was dead.

When I married their mother I felt obligated to them, just as if they were my own children. I agreed that I would treat them as my own children. The only thing I asked of them was their respect in return.

To Anita I gave the name Kakato'saakii, which is from my family. To Gilbert, when he was joining the Horn Society, I gave the name Aapspikayioohkitopi. It had belonged to his grandfather Jack Eagle Bear, who had raised him. He felt bad because his father was dead. He must have felt alone.

When a transfer is made the parents and family members are supposed to dance beside the new members of the Horn Society. He would not have his father to dance beside him. Because I now considered him as my son, I gave horses as part of the transfer payment and I did the honour announcement for him. In fact, I did the honour-announcement for a lot of the other new members. I agreed to do this for them because I had achieved the status to do so and I felt obligated.

All of my stepchildren treat me with honour and respect. Whenever I can I will help them out if they ask me. All of them visit me. Their children consider me as their grandfather and some of these want to visit me for extended periods. I talk to them too and I am giving them the benefit of my knowledge.

"You will have good luck if you do good things and you will suffer if you engage in bad behaviour," I tell them.

When I advise these young people, I encourage them to never give up, even if a challenge seems too great. "Keep trying!" I tell them. "You will eventually succeed and overcome your problems." The stories of the past people extoll this same virtue. The story of the Makoyioohsokoyi is one such example of persistence and never giving up.

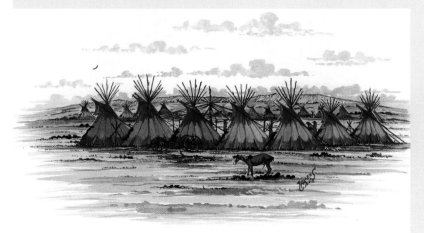

Akokatssini (Sundance) is a sacred place where Iitskinayiiksi andMao'to'kiiksi go through their annual societal ceremonies. They give special blessings to non-members who have made pledges or to those who want to have their faces painted.

GOAL(S)

1. To understand Niitsitapi spirituality.
2. To understand how nature (e.g., animals) influenced our spirituality.

OBJECTIVE(S)

1. Students will recall the story of Makoyoohsokoyi.
2. Students will discuss how the concepts of sharing, compassion, tolerance and respect were displayed in this story.
3. Students will correctly pronounce all Blackfoot terms.
4. Students will know all the meanings of Blackfoot terms used.
5. Students will correctly spell all Blackfoot terms used.

CULTURAL CONCEPT

Niitsitapiaatsimoihkaani came from nature (e.g., the animals).

STUDENT ACTIVITIES

1. Students will listen to the cultural background information as it is being read by their teacher.
2. Students in cooperative groups of four will find examples of compassion, tolerance, sharing and respect. Students will be asked to elaborate on their answers.
3. Students will report back to the class.
4. Students will invite an elder to talk about some aspect of the cultural background information.

EVALUATION ACTIVITIES

1. Students will correctly define all Blackfoot terms.
2. Students will correctly spell all Blackfoot terms.
3. Students will correctly pronounce all Blackfoot terms.
4. Students will design a quiz based on the story.
5. Students will cooperatively design a mural depicting the story.

RESOURCES

1. Various elders of Iitskinayiiksi and Mao'to'kiiksi
2. Recorded elder interviews

MAKOYOOHSOKOYI (THE WOLF TRAIL—THE MILKY WAY)

CULTURAL BACKGROUND INFORMATION

This is how Rosie Day Rider related this story.

There are many things which are holy. I am only talking now about how different people sought spirit helpers. Eagles have strong spirits. Some of the land animals that have strong powers are the beaver, otter and mink. That is why they camped together one winter. I will tell the story about this:

I had been asked about Makoyoohsokoyi (The Milky Way—The Wolf Road).

There are seven stars, Miohpokoiksi, Mamma'pisi kii nihk Ihkitsikammiksi. The stars have stories to them.

Makoyoohsokoyi is about the land animals. The time that this occurred was in the dog-days time, when the people walked everywhere. It was in the winter.

The people had been camped long in the same location. They were beginning to feel the hunger brought on by lack of fresh meat. When they were finally ready to change their camp, the bison had moved many kilometres away.

At the time they broke camp there was a lot of snow on the ground. The air was cold and the snow was deep. All the people except one man and his family moved closer to the bison herd.

The man, who did not leave with the rest, told his wives and children, "We will stay here". The reason he did this is not known. They had very little to eat. They had so little to eat there was no food for any of them.

Some wolves came to their camp and they investigated the plight of the man and his family. On their return to the animal camp, which included all the animals around, they reported: "They are very hard up. They have no more food to eat." The leader of the village told them, "You will bring this food to them," and a food pack was made ready for the man and his family.

It was night when these messengers arrived back at the small camp. When the man and his wives heard people outside they looked at each other apprehensively. "You're still home?" a voice said from outside.

"Yes," the man answered from inside his lodge. "Come in," he beckoned them. By this time the wolves had assumed human form.

Two long-chinned young men entered the lodge. "Your friend Omahkokoyi sent you this food," they told him. The man's wives jumped up and received the food that was brought. "Please do not bother feeding us. This food is meant for yourselves and your children," they told the wives. The women prepared the meat for a boiled meal.

"Tomorrow we will come back to take you to our village. Your friend Omahkokoyi has asked that you move to our camp. Pack your belongings in the morning and join us in our village where there is always plenty to eat. Our hunting is always successful."

When they left, the man asked his wives if they had noted anything strange about the two visitors. He told them that they were not real people and that there was a reason for their long pointed chins. "But we shouldn't worry about that. They have given us good food."

In the morning they made ready for their departure. This was after they had eaten the leftovers from their supper the night before. The two men arrived with others to help them move to the village. After their tipi was taken down and properly packed, the family was told to follow the men from the village.

Their journey started and was punctuated by rest stops along the way. Finally, they came over a hill. Below it was a village of many lodges. The snow had already been cleared from the location where their tipi was to be set up. No sooner had they arrived and their camp was up, complete with a warm fire inside. All they had to do was lay the bedding and other furnishings where they wanted them.

Then they heard a voice, a camp crier's voice that announced that Omahkokoyi wanted the man as his guest for a meal. He now realized that his host was the leader of the village.

Upon entering the wolf chief's lodge, he was greeted by a wonderful array of food already prepared for their eating. The man ate and informed his host that what food he could not finish, he would take with him, iimsskaaw. The chief also told him: "We invited you here not for any other reason but to help you out. We always have plenty of food. You do not even need to do any hunting."

The wolf chief told him about the other occupants of the village. Some of the animals were the black wolf, the timber wolf, the different types of foxes, the badger and the skunk. He was warned by the chief, "If the badger invites you to a meal, do not accept. They have a fatty smell about them. You will not like it. The skunk that smells even worse will probably invite you too. Do not accept that invitation as well."

Then the chief pointed to the night sky and told the man, "In the future your people will talk about that pathway in the sky," and he pointed to the Makoyoohsokoyi (Wolf Trail, Milky Way). "That is our power. Our trail will move to the sky."

Time passed and the man was invited by the different animals to meals and feasts. The day came when the badger invited him. He told his wife about the warning that he had received from the chief regarding this invitation. "I have been invited to many different camps so far and it is not right that I refuse this one." So he went.

When he entered their lodge, he noted that they were all short people. The women were not only short but they were plump as well. Their fingers were short too. They had pretty faces but they definitely had an odor about them. Every time a different animal invited the man, he was given a power by that animal. The same thing happened when he went to the badger's lodge for a feast.

He did not want to offend the badger by declining the invitation. But in order to keep his visit to a short one, he told his host shortly after he arrived, "I ate not very long ago and so I will not eat very much now. But I will pack some food for later on." He packed the food. (This practice is still going on today.) Later, when he got the food home, his wives and children did not make a fuss about the food smelling greasy. They ate it anyway. Finally, the skunk invited him. Again he felt that he could not refuse the invitation as he had accepted all the others.

They may have had odorous bodies but they were very perky creatures and moved about swiftly and deftly. Again he made the excuse that he had just eaten and that he was still full, but he would take some food for his children to eat. The skunk also gave him a sacred power, just as the other animals had done.

The man continued to live in the village and he spent much time with the wolf chief. After he had been there for a while, the chief told him, "Your people have moved back. They are not too far from here. Soon we will break up. Many of the women are pregnant and they will need to leave to give birth to their new children."

The man knew that they were not real people. But he also knew that some supernatural thing had happened which changed them temporarily into human beings.

"When the time is near for you to return to your own people, when the white part of your fingernails is very evident, that is when we will split up," the wolf chief said. The man replied, "We will miss you very much, you have been very good to us." The Wolf Chief nodded, acknowledging the kind remark. "All the sacred powers which have been transferred to you, you will keep. You now have the power to use them, they are yours. You will take them home with you." The animals had not only saved him and his family from starvation, they had bestowed all of their individual powers to him.

These powers and gifts that he received were the basis for our societies and everything that we consider sacred.

Then the wolf chief warned him: "Listen very carefully to what I am about to tell you. The time is coming very quickly when the single men will become very agitated. They will act strangely and wildly. It may pique your interest to find out what is happening outside, but do not try to look out. Later on, when the commotion is over and you come outside, you will see things lying on the ground. Do not touch anything."

Soon, true to what the wolf chief had foretold, the day came when the single men of the animal people went into a frenzy. The man and his family heard a big commotion in the village. They saw the outlines of bodies fall against the wall of their tipi and they heard many excited voices. "We must mind our own business and not try to find out what is going on outside," he told his wife and children. They did not even go near the door of their lodge for a peek outside.

Eventually, the volume of the noise outside subsided and a lull returned to the village. They went outside. One of his children, a boy, noticed an arrow on the ground. Because children are very curious people, he ran to the arrow and picked it up without thinking.

As soon as he picked it up, the arrow turned into wolf dung and a collective howl from all the animals was heard. Then they scattered and ran from the village.

Earlier, when the wolf chief had been giving instructions to the man, he had also told him what to do when all the animals scattered. Now he and his family collected all the food from the village. All the meat, the stores of berries, and the hides from the many successful hunts the animal people had had were collected. All the herbs, roots and other medicines were also collected.

The man and his family continued to live by themselves for a little while. Great was the feeling of loneliness they felt with the animal people all gone. Then the great warm chinook blew in and spring arrived. When this happened, the lone family rejoined their village.

This is what we were given. This is how Niitsitapiaatsimoihkaani began.

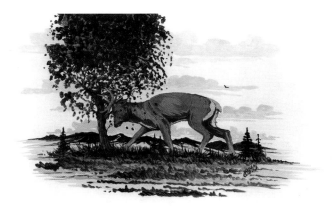

Some of Niitsitapiaatsimoihkaani came from the animal world.

HOW KSIMMOTSIISINI (MILD VERBAL DERISION) HELPED TO DETERMINE THE NAMES OF THE THREE BLACKFOOT-SPEAKING TRIBES OF ALBERTA AND MONTANA

GOAL(S)

1. To understand how ksimmotsiisini determined the names of the three Blackfoot-speaking tribes of Alberta and Montana.
2. To raise student self-esteem.

OBJECTIVE(S)

1. Students will retell how ksimmotsiisini gave the Kainai, the Siksika and the Piikani tribes their tribal names.
2. Students will explain what ksimmotsiisini is.
3. Students will learn what tolerance is.
4. Students will explain how their practice influenced behaviour.

CULTURAL CONCEPT

Ksimmotsiisini determined what names the Blackfoot-speaking tribes gave to each other.

STUDENT ACTIVITIES

1. In cooperative groups of four, students will discuss ksimmotsiisini.
2. Students will talk to their grandparents and ask them about ksimmotsiisini and bring back examples. They will share these with the class.
3. Students will pretend that the communities of Standoff, Levern and Moses Lake have split off from the Blood Reserve. They give each other names. What names would they give to each of these communities? Give reasons why these names were chosen.

EVALUATION ACTIVITIES

1. Students will write a short paper on ksimmotsiisini, explaining the practice.
2. Students will bring in examples of ksimmotsiisini.
3. Students will ask their grandparents about two people who practice ksimmonisiisini on each other.

RESOURCES

1. Elders from school lists
2. *Kitomahkitapiiminnooniksi— Stories from Our Elders*, Vol. 1–3 Flora Zaharia and Leo Fox

HOW KSIMMOTSIISINI (MILD VERBAL DERISION) HELPED TO DETERMINE THE NAMES OF THE THREE BLACKFOOT-SPEAKING TRIBES OF ALBERTA AND MONTANA

CULTURAL BACKGROUND INFORMATION

Up to a certain time in the past, the Kainai, Piikani and Siksika were one nation. Our ancestors spoke a common language and shared a common culture. Through intermarriage and adoption the three tribes were linked together.

When they separated, Siksikawa moved northward. Among all the relatives, it was the men who took a leadership role. Kainaiwa remained here. Piikaniwa moved toward the Heart Butte area. It was as if there was a fence around our common territory to keep strangers from coming in.

With the breakup of the one nation into three separate tribes came the practice of ksimmotsiisini (mild verbal derision). One tribe always had to be "better" than the other two. Each tribe also liked to make fun of the other two.

According to the story told, two things contributed to how the Siksika got their name.

One was the colour of the soil. The Siksika lived in an area where the soil was quite dark. Every time they walked or ran anywhere, they had to walk or run over this dark soil. Each time they did this, their moccasins would become darker and dirtier than the last time.

If they could have washed their moccasins to keep them clean, no doubt they would have ended up with another name. But all they could do was rub the leather together to try and dislodge the discolouring dirt. The fact that they could not wash their moccasins was the second factor which contributed to how they got their name— "…siksikawa. Moi iimayai siksikawa." (…black feet. Those people who have such black feet.) Because it was used frequently, the name of Siksikai'tsitapii (Blackfoot People) became commonly accepted.

We turn now to the Piikani. It is said about the Piikani that their women have always enjoyed more freedom from household duties than the women of the other two tribes. Piikani women could be leaders in their tribe. It is still like this even to the present time. Because of this, the men were not strict with their women in how well they did their household chores.

Generally speaking, a man of wealth in those days had many wives, and the perception was that these wives were like servants. It was because of these women that a man had a tipi to live in, and this was kept clean. It was also the wives who organized the storing and preparation of the food. They fed the man. Whenever there was a successful hunt, it was the women who looked after the skinning of the buffalo and the preparation of the meat for drying. It was also the women's job to tan the hide.

Among the Piikani (as the story goes), life was not so well organized, and it showed. One way it showed was in their hide tanning. Their hides showed many imperfections. They looked like they were dirty, even when they were freshly tanned. Because of the lack of attention to detail, there were many spots on these hides which looked as if the animals had been in a sickly condition before they were killed.

Eventually, the other two tribes began to refer to them as "mooksi iimaawaapikaniiwa… moi aapikaniiwa." (Those people with the scabby robes, the scabby-robed people). Just as in the case of the Siksika, the name came into common usage and was shortened to "Piikani."

Then it was the other tribe's turn to respond in kind to us. Because we were all chiefs when they talked about us, they would preface their remarks with "moi kanainaway, moi mo'toinaway." (The all-chiefs people, where all the people are chiefs.) There were variations of this over time until eventually we were "Kainai." Aapaiaitsitapi, which is our other name, was usurped by this new name.

RECORDING HISTORY THROUGH THE WINTER COUNT AND STORYTELLING

GOAL(S)	OBJECTIVE(S)	CULTURAL CONCEPT
1. To understand what the winter count was. 2. To understand the role of storytellers. 3. To understand the difference between oral and written history.	1. Students will differentiate between oral and written history. 2. Students will discuss why storytellers are important to the tribe. 3. Students will understand how winter counts worked.	The winter count and storytelling were important in keeping oral history accurate.

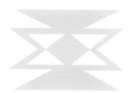

STUDENT ACTIVITIES	EVALUATION ACTIVITIES	RESOURCES
1. In groups of four, have the students develop "winter counts" for the last five years. 2. Have a class discussion about their "winter counts." 3. Have the students interview elders and find out why the practice of storytelling has virtually stopped. What were some of the factors which led to this? How did these factors impact on the practice? 4. Have each student bring in his or her mother's name or father's name in Blackfoot. Have each student explain the meaning of these names. 5. Have the students discuss their names and why they were given. Discuss why some people have so many names.	1. Have the students illustrate a family winter count using important events in their family histories. 2. Have each students "storytell" their family winter count. 3. Have each student research and write a two-page paper on actual examples of winter counts. 4. Have each student find out the protocol of a name-giving ceremony. For those who do not have a Blackfoot name, have a name-giving ceremony at a special school assembly.	1. Kainai elders on school lists 2. Libraries at Red Crow Community College, Kainai High School, Tatsikiisaapo'p Middle School, Levern Elementary School, Saipoyi Elementary School, Ninastako Cultural Centre and the University of Lethbridge

RECORDING HISTORY THROUGH THE WINTER COUNT AND STORYTELLING

CULTURAL BACKGROUND INFORMATION

Roughly defined, history is all the events which have taken place in the past. The form of history which we use in school today is written history. Important events which had an impact on people and the societies in which these people lived were recorded on paper and most often bound into books. This written history was transferred from one generation to the next generation in this manner.

In order for people to record these events on paper, they needed a system of writing. The English language has a writing system or orthography which includes twenty-six letters. French and Spanish are similar. The writing system of these societies enabled them to record their histories.

By the time the Anglo-Europeans arrived in North America, no writing system had been devised by our ancestors. Some First Nations wrote down important information in caves or on the side of mountains using symbols and depictions of animals and people. The Kainai, Siksika and Piikani used what has been termed the winter count to record each year. The winter count depicted the most outstanding event which took place in a particular year.

Since there was more than one person who made these recordings, the outstanding events could be different. For example, if there had been a year when a solar eclipse took place, and this was considered by one recorder as the outstanding event of that year, then he would record this. In the same year, another historian might have recorded something different, for example, many deaths caused by a terrible winter storm. The end result was the same. When reference was made to either of these events, the people would realize that they were talking about the same year. In fact, two important events were recorded.

The winter count served as a chronological measure of time. Other tribal history was transferred from one generation to the next by oral history. This kind of history was memorized history. It was repeated by individuals at storytelling sessions when people visited each other. As happens so often, some individuals developed more skill in this, and this was noted. As the history was passed on to others, and it was repeated by a listener, reference would be made to the skilled aitsinikii (storyteller). He would say, at the end of his repetition of the story, "This is how the story was told to me by …" In this manner, the people were able to keep an accurate record of events.

In the 1950s, this was still being done by skilled storytellers. In the decade which followed, the practice began to decline precipitously because the older generation was dying off. The decline has kept on until today. There may only be a handful of these storytellers left. Listed by all of their Blood First Nation names are some of the last of the skilled storytellers: Saisikka'pii also known as Kiaayisttsomo'kii also known as John Fox (1907–1982); Atsi'tsiina also known as Piitaisaapo'p also known as Mia'nistohkitopi also known as Omahksisttsiiksiinaikoan also known as Aokitsikinii also known as Willy Eagle Plume (1907–1976); Ksaahkomm also known as Naato'siina also known as Alfred Eagle Plume (1903–1990); and lkkimaani also known as Jim Bottle (1904–1981).

RESIDENTIAL SCHOOL INTERVIEW

ELDER/SURVIVOR D

I went to school at St. Paul's from 1943 to about 1949. Our parents knew that we had to go to school and that is why they sent us. St. Paul's Anglican Indian Residential School was the only school that we could attend.

1943–1949

We had reading, arithmetic, science and writing. We also had religious classes. These religious classes were held in the morning and in the evening in the chapel. I did not find what I learned in school useful later on. But I did learn some English.

At home, before I went to school, we spoke Blackfoot all the time. That was my first language. When I went to school, I could not use this language anymore. If I did, I got punished. The supervisor would get very upset. She would slap us on the mouth. We were also made to stand in the hallway for a lengthy period. Sometimes, some students got the strap.

I was happy in the intermediate class. The teacher was very nice to me. She was a nice person. We got to sing.

But the school was bad in more ways than it was good. The food, for example, was bad. So was the way we were treated. We were also forced to work for half a day. We never got to finish our school work because we had to work. And if we didn't do this work right, we were hit with the cleaner cans and forced to start all over again.

It is good to be able to pray in the Indian way. It helps to pray for everybody. It is good to help people out. I still pray sometimes in the Christian way, but I am more involved with our cultural ways now.

I suffered abuse in the residential school. Once, the supervisor broke a yardstick because he kept hitting me and hitting me. Another girl had to stand in front of the playroom with a clothes pin on her tongue. Some of the other students cried for her. We were all upset by this.

I hated school. Many nights I cried myself to sleep. It was a lonely experience. We were treated like we were in the army.

ELDER/SURVIVOR E

1950–1951

1959–1960

I must have been about nine years old when I went to school. I was sick. I had rheumatic fever. I went to St. Mary's Indian Residential School. The years that I spent there were from about 1950–51 to 1959–60.

The priest recruited me. When they thought it was time for you to go to school they would come around. They may have threatened my dad. I had to attend St. Mary's. It was either there or St. Paul's but my dad was a Roman Catholic.

We were taught the basic things because the government didn't really want us to learn. It was just basic reading and writing and, of course, housework.

The teaching was useful when I left school. I learned to be a good parent and a good housekeeper. It caused me to encourage my kids to go further in school because of what little I got.

When I went to school I spoke only Blackfoot. I always got a red star because I spoke Blackfoot. My grandparents did not speak English. My grandmother only used English when she swore. We were discouraged from using Blackfoot while we were in school. We were punished if we spoke it.

I saw others punished for speaking Blackfoot. I was never really punished for speaking it because my grandparents always visited me and they knew what happened to me. I always reported if anything bad happened to me.

A gold star meant that you were a good girl, that you spoke mostly English in the playroom.

The ones with red stars got punished. They could not go to a movie and they had to go to bed early.

This was done in the playrooms, not in the classroom.

We reported everything bad to our parents or grandparents. Many students did this. Then we got punished too for reporting these things home.

But something good came from this. I learned to be a good parent. I think I was more stable when I became a parent than some young parents today. I also learned to become a good Christian. I made a lot of friends in school—young and old. Because I was raised by my grandparents, I knew how to get along with all kinds of people. I learned how to be a good housekeeper.

Because the food was bad, we were always starving, we were always hungry. We ate very simple meals, only one slice of bread, porridge, soup. The only time we ate really well was when the bishop came. We only got some butter to put on our bread on Sunday.

Traditional Indian religion/spirituality is really good. We're a lot closer to the Creator. We try to be better every day.

I still practice some of the things I learned in residential school but my husband has really turned around. He has gone totally Indian religion.

Sometimes I say the rosaries. I have combined Catholicism and Indian religion. The two are very similar. However, there are some differences. For example, in our own spirituality, it is up to us to forgive ourselves and try to do better next time, whereas in the Roman Catholic, you seek forgiveness by going to confession and getting forgiveness from a priest.

One time we got a strap because we all slept together, all the senior girls. We were just telling each other stories, we were not doing anything bad. All of us got a strap. I got strapped twice because I would not cry.

I used to see some of the students get abused by some supervisors and some teachers. There were two girls who were in my class who suffered this kind of abuse. One girl was very shy; she would not speak up. The other girl was very slow; she couldn't remember things for very long. They were repeatedly strapped by the teacher for this.

Then there were some girls who were awful bullies. They used to make life miserable for some of the more timid girls.

There was one nun supervisor who was very mean. I remember one girl who was repeatedly hit so many times by this nun she peed in her pants.

I was even bit by one teacher's dog and nothing was done about it.

We could not look at the boys when we went downstairs to eat. If we did we were punished and we were told that we were sinning.

I was sixteen going on seventeen when I left school. One of the reasons I ran away with my first husband was because I did not want to go back to school.

We were given numbers rather than our names in the playrooms.

I remember one of the girls saying that the visiting dentist had been feeling her body. She reported this. However, instead of something being done to the dentist, this girl was punished.

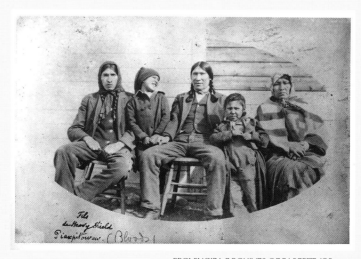

PROVINCIAL ARCHIVES OF ALBERTA/OB.9057

Heavy Shield and his family.

ELDER/SURVIVOR F

1948

When I was seven years old I went to school at St. Mary's Indian Residential School. I wanted to go to school because I thought there was a lot of fun there. Little did I realize what was ahead of me.

An older cousin tried to warn me as he had already gone to school. "Don't go to school," he told me. But I didn't want to listen to him. When I walked into the building for the first time, I knew I had made a mistake.

My dad wanted me to go to St. Mary's, even though my mother didn't want me to go there. I got scared the first time I walked into the school, with all those Grey Nuns walking around.

We prayed a lot. I think we were more or less forced to pray a lot but that helped me. Today I'm still a Catholic and I'm proud of it. I'm not against our own Indian religion. I just don't get involved in it.

The discipline was very strict at residential school. For some this was abusive. I used to run away from school because I was lonely for my parents. I ran away twice and I got strapped for these but I reported them to my parents. I didn't wait. My mother had told the priest not to strap me when he came to pick me up but I got strapped anyway. She later came to the school to check on me and when she found out I had been strapped, she got after the priest.

I remember some of the punishment that was given out for talking in church. We either had to wash the toilets or we had to wash the stairs.

When I first went to school, I don't recall being told not to speak Blackfoot. But in 1956 or 1957, I remember that there were rewards for those students who spoke English. I remember once they got to go to a movie. The supervisor had reported that I was not one of the ones who spoke English so I was left behind. I was about fifteen years old then. Now the opposite is true.

After one of the times I ran away from school, I was kept inside on November 11. There was no school that day. The other students went for a walk or a hike along the Bull Horn. That was the only treat for the day. Myself, a cousin of mine and an older boy were locked in the small boys' room. Even the washroom was locked to us. We could not use it if we had to. One of the other boys had to pee. He did.

One of the supervisors was mean to this boy who was a little slow. One time we were doing some exercises in the gym and this boy could not do what he was supposed to do. The supervisor grabbed him and threw him on the floor.

I don't think this is sexual abuse but one time the supervisor had to examine us to check for disease, scabs and stuff like that. After we showered we went one by one into his room where we took off all of our clothes and he examined us. This inspection was very thorough because he lifted our genitals this way and that to examine us.

I don't agree with the lawsuit which is going on now against the residential schools. If these people were abused, why did they wait so long to bring it up? They probably lived badly because of it. If they were sick with it why didn't they bring it up earlier instead of living with it day after day, year after year? Now most of the people involved are dead. If healing is involved, you heal yourself. Be strong and heal yourself. You don't need others to heal you.

When I was in school, if the nuns or priests did anything to me I told my parents right away. My mother was Anglican and she did not hesitate to speak up for me against the priests and nuns.

I remember this one girl who was very slow. She was punished because she could not do her school work. She was strapped. This might have been physical abuse.

The level of education we got was pretty low. One of the reasons was because many of the nuns could not speak proper English. We learned to speak English with their French Canadian accent. The Anglicans spoke better English than we did.

Of course nitsiikattsissk in school. I didn't really apply myself to learn. The Grey Nuns taught me in grades one and two. In grade three I got this regular teacher who was very good to me. I learned a lot from her. I think she taught me for three years.

I went as far as grade eleven. I spent fifteen years in school. All of them were in residential school. I had to repeat some grades.

Some families were experiencing hardship, that is why some children were placed in residential school. They not only got food but also some education. There were also some children who were more or less raised by the nuns and priests.

I don't ever recall a parent coming into the school to complain to a priest or nun that we were being taught too much religion and not enough regular education.

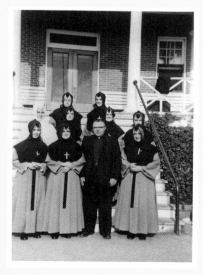

St. Mary's Residential School, 1958.

GEORGE FIRST RIDER

Oki nistowakao'k Matoomohkitopiwa. Anohkai ihkanitaihtsiw sopo'wahtsi'sini. Kiannohkai nitsiitsinikokoiyi, iikakaitapi mooksi omahkitapiiksi aitsinikiiksi. Kianohk aamoksk omahksimmiksi issksinimmi annoom matapiiwa, Siksikawa, Kainaiwa, Aamskaapipikaniiwa ihkanai'tokskao'p isskoohtsik. Kaatohkanawa'sokitapiiyio'p anohk.

Aakaaatahsi kiikahtominnoona

kiistonnoona stamitohkanaoksinaop anno ksahkoiyi. Anohk ksiistsikoihk iimanistaipaitapiiyio'p. Maatsitstsipa aahksikkahsistotooki. Amo Siksikawa stamohkanawaapatohsisttotsiw. Mooksi kayio'kowammotsiiksi ninaiksi o'totama'psi. Annoom Kainaiwa noom stamita'pai'tapiiw. Ammoi stamohkatsitapowa oiskitsipahpiistak.Anno, ammoi miiksistohtsistsiipisskato'p naamitapiiwa mahkitsito'tohsi.

Oki, ksiiimmotsiisini, a'panisttsiisini, annioyaok ai'tstsiw.

Aohpokawahkaotsiima matapiiwa mo Piikaniwa ki noo Kainaiwa ki ma Siksikawa. Anno Kainaiwa sootamaisskahsaisskitstaaw.

Stamaisskahsaisskitstaw mii okahtomsini. Mooksi kaatohkanaya'tammi anohk amoksi kaahtomiinaiksi.

Aamsskaapohta iitamitsa'tam mohk Osaohkowahk.Hann. Kii no kiistonnoona Iikaisskiniiyiawa,iitohkanaya'tammiaw.

Oki anohkai mii ksiimmotsiisini, sayiiksiksaapsini kiistonnoona aawattsinihkattsiiyio'p. Moi Siksiksawa. Ma Siksikawayia otsikahkohsi mi annia naanistoohtsim otsikahkohsi mii. Annaak aikakoohkapssonnim otsistotoohsiistsi maataissiiststaawa aikakaipssonnimai. Aanistsa'po'si ma matapiw mo sikahkoiyi aitsikainattsii matsikiistsi. Sootamohtsinihkataw moi Siksikawa. "Siksikawa, moi iimayaisiksikaway." Maatamiwa miistsi ohkattowawaistsi. Miistsi matsikiowawaistsi annistsiyiok matsoowawaistsi aitsikainamm. Nainayita'tam "Siksikay, Siksikaitsitapi."

Oki amoi Aamskaapipikaniwa. Aania'siwa anohk ksiistsikoihk iimainaimatsiwa otohkiimaaniksi. Ainao'kiimawa. Sootamsawayiiksskoiyi otohkiimaiksi ma ota'po'takihsini. Naak matapiiwa ihtawaakaohkiimiw omiiksistsahkomaapiim miiksi otohkiimaiksi. Anniksiyio'kiaiksi ihtaohkookoiyiiyiawaiksi, ihtaohkoinstawaopiiyiaw, ihtaohkooyiitapiw. Otayiisookiawaiksi, otaoiyiistotookiawaiksi, otaikkiahkaanistomookiawaiksi otohko'tsimaanowawaistsi iinii. Oki ma Aamskaapipikaniiwa stamsohtsa'piiw opaitapiisini. Miiksi Aamskaapitapiiksi maaaiwawaiksi aohkanawaapikaniinammiaw, aikanainamm, miaawaistsi aawaapikanii. Annooksi stamohkattsipo'tainihkatsiiyiawaiksi "mooksi iimawaapikaniiw. Moi aapikaniiwa. Naanawai aapikaniwa'siw kianohk ksiistsikoihk iimiitaihtsiw Piikani. Oomiksi otohkiimaanowawaiksi otsowayiika'po'takihsaw.

Oki oostowaway nohkitsipo'tsatsipssakkiiyiaw. Taka noom kanainaw, noom. Stamaniiw "Moi kanainaway, moi mo'toinaway, moi mo'toinaway." Niita'payiohkiitsiw naanowai Kainaiwa'so'p. Aok anohkayi anniyiok mii a'panisttspi "Kainai." Anohk ksiistsikoi aitsstsinihka'siimato'p. A'tamiaapi'powa'siw "Kainai." Mi kitsinihka'sinnooni "Aapai'tsitapi," kitohkanai'tsinihka'sinnoon "Aapai'tsitapi" aahtsowai'saipo'tsi'p ki saakiitainihkakkiiyiaw naapiikoaiksi, saakiainihkatoomiaw "Blood Indians." Kianohkai aahtsowayaissiinihp mi "Aapai'tsitapi" ki mii stamitotoomihtsiw "Kainai." Ki anohkay issksinihki aanistapiww i'powattsiisin ihtsi Kainaiwa'so'p.

Kianohkayi ma Aamskaapipikaniiwa otaotayamoohsi mooksi matapiiksi.Niistowa nitssksinowa aamohk aanistawahk Aisstoyiimsta, anno i'tsiistsipihtaw otohkiimaan anistsyini Ksisstoyi'tsimaan. Stamitsstsitapisttotsiw Piikani. Kianohk iitsi'niw Piikani. Aamoi Aapatohsipikaniiwa kaatsitohkanaissksahkomiw Aamskaapohtsi. Annikai to'tsiw. Anniai nistapiw moohk niinihka'simi. Hann.

Stamitsstsitapisttotsiw Piikani kianohk iitsi'niw Piikani. Aamoi Aapatohsipikaniiwa kaatsitohkanaissksahkomiw Aamskaapohtsi annikai to'tsiw. Anniai nistapiw mohk niinihka'simi. Hann.

History of the Blackfoot Speaking Tribes

Oki, my name is [George] First Rider. Questions are always being asked now. The stories that I know were told to me by a lot of elders. Today, the older people know that about our people, the Siksikawa, Kainaiwa, Aamskaapipikaniiwa, we were all one nation in the past. That is why we are all mixed today. When we went to war, it is believed that we were the meanest in the land. To this day we are still here. No one got the best of us.

The Siksika moved north. All the people who were related went. The men were the leaders in their clans. The Kainai remained here. The [Piikani] moved toward Heart Butte. This is how a virtual fence was created around our territory so that strangers could not move in.

The practice of one-upmanship and making fun of each other came into existence. The people of Piikani and Kainai and Siksika all fought together against their enemies. Kainai always seemed to display the most bravery of the three. Our tribe always seemed to show the most bravery in war. That is why our war leaders were so prominent. The only prominent war leader among the Piikani was Osaohko. Here, Iikaisskini was only one among many.

Because of the practice of one-upmanship and making fun of each other, we gave each other names. In the case of Siksika, I heard that the dark colour of the earth there had something to do with how they got their name.

In those days the people did not wash their clothes. They just tried to remove the dirt as best they could by rubbing and shaking the hide. Whenever the people went outside, the dark earth would stain their mocassins and their leggings. "They have black feet," said the other people. Over time the name stuck and the people were called Siksika. It was not their actual feet being black—it was their mocassins and their leggings. They became known as Siksika, Siksikai'tsitapii.

Then there was the Piikani. It is said today that women among the Peigan are still the chiefs. It is like the men marry chiefs. Their expectations of their women, as far as work was concerned, were not too high. In the past the people had many wives because of necessity. Their wives were almost like hired employees. These wives made the lodges, they kept them clean, they provided a home. These women served the food, they cooked and they dressed whatever buffalo meat was secured. The southern Piikani lagged behind in this practice. Consequently, their robes looked rough, like they had scabs on them. The people described this characteristic about their appearance when they talked about the Piikani saying, "Mooksi iimawaapikaniw, moi aapikaniiwa." Over time and usage, they came to be known as Piikani. It was because their women did not work very hard.

Then it was the other people's turn to describe us. We thought we were all chiefs here. When other people talked about us, they would say, when referring to us, "Moi kanainaway, moi mo'toinaway, moi mo'toinaway." The name varied here and there until finally we were Kainai. It was because of talk that we got this name. To this day we are known by this name—we are even called that in English. Our name, our collective name of Aapai'tsitapii, is being left out, even though some white people still call us Blood Indians. Aapai'tsitapii is being replaced by Kainai.

Then it was the breakaway group from the southern Piikani. I knew the man called Aisstoyiimsta who eloped here with his new wife Ksisstoyi'tsimaan. He never returned home but kept going until he settled with the Piikani north of here. This is the reason why so many northern Piikani own land in the United States.

This is the story behind the names.

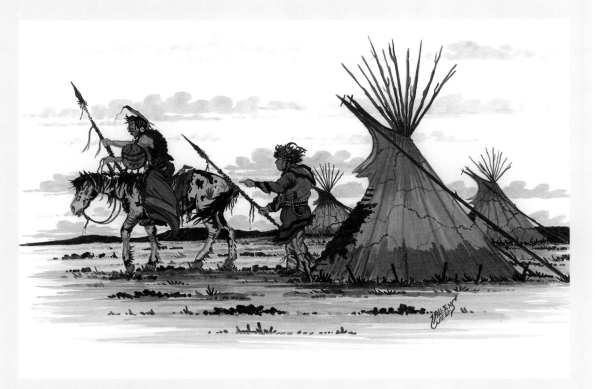

Ni'taitsskaiksi – Lone fighters clan

A TRADITIONAL NIITSITAPI MARRIAGE

7

GOAL(S)

To understand the traditional Niitsitapi marriage.

OBJECTIVE(S)

1. Students will describe how a traditional Niitsitapi marriage was arranged.
2. Students will explain why the practice of having multiple wives was established.
3. Students will describe the punishment carried out against those women who refused to comply with their parent's wishes in arranged marriages.
4. Students will explain how respect influenced the behaviour of a man and his mother–in-law. Also, how respect affected the behaviour of a young single woman.

CULTURAL CONCEPT

The traditional Niitsitapi marriage was arranged by a young woman's parents. The greatest consideration was the well-being of the young woman after marriage.

STUDENT ACTIVITIES

1. Students will listen to the cultural background information as it is read by the teacher or another student.
2. Students in cooperative groups of four will do a creative writing exercise where a short story is developed using the cultural background information. Students will share their stories when they are completed.
3. Students will compare and contrast traditional and modern marriage practices.
4. Students will put themselves in the place of a young bride or prospective husband in a traditional marriage and write about their feelings. These can be shared with the class when they are completed.

EVALUATION ACTIVITIES

1. Students will critically discuss the following:
a) How did parents choose a husband for their daughter?
b) The practice of multiple wives.
c) The shunning which occurred between a man and his mother-in-law.
2. Students will write a short critical essay on arranged marriages.

RESOURCES

1. Kainai elders
2. Taped elder interviews
3. *Kitomahkitapiiminnooniksi– Stories from Our Elders,* Vol. 1–3

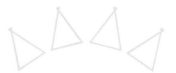

A TRADITIONAL NIITSITAPI MARRIAGE

CULTURAL BACKGROUND INFORMATION

When she was considered to be the right age for marriage, a young woman's parents met with an elder and they consulted with this person about the right mate for their daughter. They met not so much to find a young man but to reassure themselves that the one they wanted had the desired traits they valued. Was this young man as resourceful as he seemed to be? Was he as kind as they believed he was?

When they were reassured, the old man went to the lodge of the parents of the young man. "Are you home?" he called out when he arrived. "Apiit (come in)," he was told. The parents of the young man suspected the reason for his visit. Then the elder, who in reality was a marriage broker, informed them of the reason for his visit. They talked.

Maybe the young man was still single, or maybe he already had a wife or two. In any case, his parents listened respectfully to the elder. "It's alright. It sounds good," they would say. So they agreed to the marriage proposal. Then they asked that a day be set for the union.

When this was done, the women of the girl's clan went into a frenzy of preparation for the event. Moccasins for their future son-in-law had to be made. A tipi with all the furnishings had to be sewn and made ready. Extra food had to be put together to accompany the young woman into her marriage. When everything was ready she was moved to the location of her future husband's clan.

Once the bride reached her destination, the members of her entourage quickly set up her tipi. If there was a sacred object which came with the tipi, a ceremony was necessary to bless both the young woman and her husband so that they could be around this sacred object. Once this blessing was done they were considered to be married. Then, the groom's people also gave presents to the young bride.

In the rare event that a girl refused to agree to the wishes of her parents to marry whom they had chosen, she would have the tip of her nose or a finger cut off. This mark of her disobedience would remain with her for the rest of her life. Because of this, it was rare that a girl refused. All the girls knew the consequences of disagreeing to go through with an arranged union.

In many instances, unmarried sisters were married to the same man when they came of age to marry. Because of his success in the hunt and in providing well for his family, the parents of the women believed such marriages would ensure the well-being of their children. All of these wives worked together to help their common husband. Also, they joined together in raising any child born to one of them. There was a sharing of responsibilities.

The practice of having two wives is not that far into the past.

A mother could not come face to face with her son-in-law. Aisstoyiisattsiimiiwai. If she happened to see him coming, she would change her route to avoid meeting him. This was still being practiced in the 1930s and 1940s. When a son-in-law happened to be in the home of his in-laws, his wife's mother would be in a corner covered by a shawl. He would quickly do what he was there to do and then leave again. Even today in more traditional families there are remnants of this practice between a mother-in-law and her daughter's husband.

This practice was a sign of respect. In the past, girls did not engage in sex until they were married. If an unmarried girl even tried to speak of sex in a joking manner, she was severely reprimanded by her parents or older relatives. The practice of aisstoyiisattsi was part of the respect for sexual privacy between two adult individuals.

GOAL(S)	OBJECTIVE(S)	CULTURAL CONCEPT
To understand why there were rules for the pregnant woman.	1. Students will discuss the rules a pregnant woman had to follow and the reasoning behind each one. 2. Students will compare and contrast these rules with today and evaluate their validity.	In traditional Kainai society a pregnant woman had to follow certain rules. These rules were there to protect her future child.

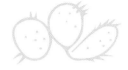 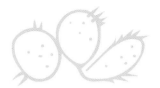

STUDENT ACTIVITIES	EVALUATION ACTIVITIES	RESOURCES
1. Students will interview a woman elder and ask her to elaborate on the rules for pregnancy. 2. Students will interview a health nurse and discuss the traditional rules with her. They will compare traditional rules with modern practices. 3. In cooperative groups of four, students will design posters depicting the rules. These will be presented to the Health Centre.	1. Students will correctly divide the rules into the categories of: a) cultural rules b) health rules. 2. Students will research the "health" rules and validate them.	1. Women elders like Rosie Day Rider, Margaret Hindman, Louise Crop Eared Wolf, Rosie Red Crow, health nurses, health care workers

HOW A WOMAN WAS PREPARED FOR CHILDBIRTH

CULTURAL BACKGROUND INFORMATION

When a girl was pregnant, her in-laws helped to prepare her for the birth of her child.

The term was, "ai'psstsikoyiisiw" which meant, "the fluid entered her." Now the term that is commonly used is "aistsi'tsaana'psiw," which means "she is in a delicate way."

When she was pregnant she was instructed on what she should and what she should not eat. She was told to do a lot of walking around, to not become sedentary. They believed this movement helped to circulate the blood in her system, thus ensuring that the fetus was healthy. When she needed to assume a different sleeping position at night, she was also instructed to do it in the safest way. Abrupt movements were to be avoided. One of the reasons for doing this was that it prevented the fetus from tying its umbilical chord around itself in the womb.

If someone in the community died and there was a corpse, the pregnant woman was warned not to look at it. It was believed that her future child would be a crying child if the mother did this. The pregnant woman learned to heed the advice given to her and she looked after her body.

She was told also never to stand in the entryway of a lodge but to completely come out of it. The belief was that the child inside her would follow her example when it was ready to come out. If she did otherwise, the child might only show its head and delay bringing the rest of its body out.

There were a lot of rules which a pregnant woman had to heed.

Older women, probably in groups of three, prepared the woman for delivery. They prepared potions which helped in the smooth delivery of the child. They also restrained the woman during the delivery. Later, they cut the umbilical chord and wrapped up the newborn child.

The new mother nursed her child soon after birth. She was discouraged from lying down and sleeping. Her blood circulation was important.

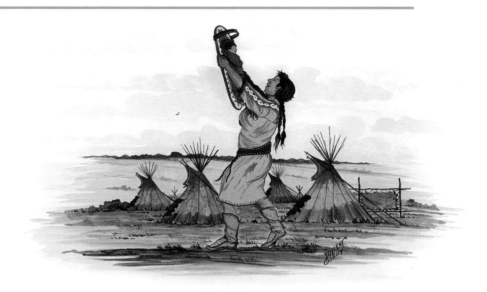

When a mother holds her new relative for the first time, she feels as if she is standing on top of the world.

GOAL(S)	OBJECTIVE(S)	CULTURAL CONCEPT
To understand that children from a very early age were taught the skills associated with their gender.	1. Students will discuss the process of how children in traditional society were instructed from early childhood to puberty. 2. Students will discuss how gender determined what would be taught to children.	Niitsitapi children were shown how to fulfill their roles from early childhood on. This process was life-long.

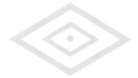

STUDENT ACTIVITIES	EVALUATION ACTIVITIES	RESOURCES
1. Students will have a class discussion on the information presented. 2. Students will compare and contrast this information with their own experiences. They will work in cooperative groups of four to do this (15 minutes). 3. Students will report back to the class by groups.	1. Students will design a quiz with their cooperative groups and give this test to another group until all students have scored perfectly. 2. Students will design a poster in their cooperative groups using graphics to illustrate how children learned in traditional society.	1. Kainai elders: Rosie Day Rider, Rosie Red Crow, Bruce Wolf Child, Adam Delaney 2. Recorded interviews of elders—*Kitomahkitapiiminnooniksi*

CULTURAL BACKGROUND INFORMATION

Hospitality was greatly emphasized. Looking after a visitor, making him feel welcome immediately, was important. Giving him something to drink and something to eat shortly after his arrival was paramount in this hospitality.

"Come in. Sit over there," a guest would be told. The girl learned to welcome people into her home.

She also learned to gather foods like berries when the time was right. She learned how they were cooked. Also, how they were dried and prepared for storage was another responsibility.

Her mother and grandmothers all had the responsibility of ensuring that she learned the skills considered to be a woman's skills. Her teachers did not hesitate to correct her when she was not doing the right thing.

THE INDOCTRINATION OF BOYS

The father was responsible for teaching his sons about the ways of men. This included the art of hunting. Because the weather influenced the hunt, studying nature and forecasting the weather was another skill taught to a young boy.

Of great importance in this education was the care of horses. After it was first brought here around 1750, this animal achieved an important status in a very short time. The best grazing area around an encampment had to be determined. This location had to have access to water and be strategically located in case of an attack by unfriendly tribes.

Which horses to break for riding and pulling had to be determined. The actual method of breaking a horse and training it were paramount in this education. This also included the building of holding pens for the animal. The boy stuck with his father and learned as much as he could.

Included in these lessons were those which transmitted the social culture. Showing proper respect for elders and tribal customs was included in this teaching. The men tried to impart in their sons all the knowledge necessary to lead a good life which followed tribal customs.

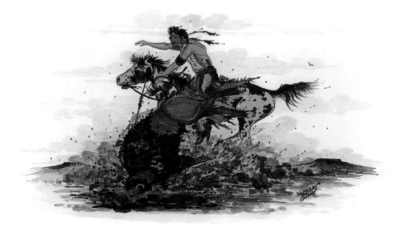

The man's role in the past was to hunt and secure food for his family and clan.

GOAL(S)

1. To understand that each member of the traditional extended family had a role.
2. To understand that a traditional leader led by example.
3. To understand that nature played a great part in the traditional extended family.

OBJECTIVE(S)

1. Students will list the responsibilities of each member of the extended family.
2. Students will explain that a leader acquired his leadership through feats in war, his kindness and his generosity.
3. Students will determine the number of leaders in the tribe by the number of clans.
4. Students will discuss how nature influenced the roles of the traditional extended family.
5. Students will discuss how children's play mimicked adult behaviour and how this influenced their later adult lives.

CULTURAL CONCEPT

Each member of the traditional extended family had a role to play. Nature influenced these roles.

STUDENT ACTIVITIES

1. Students will listen as cultural background information is given.
2. Students in cooperative groups of four will discuss the various roles of extended family members. They will prepare a chart comparing and contrasting this with the modern nuclear family. Students will report to the class in their groups.
3. Students will research the practice of multiple wives among other cultural groups and will report their findings to the class. This research will be done in cooperative groups of four.

EVALUATION ACTIVITIES

1. Students will correctly list at least two roles of each extended family member in a quiz.
2. Cooperative groups of four will design a test using the information provided.

RESOURCES

1. Elders
2. Taped elder interviews
3. *Blackfoot Lodge Tales*

ROLES IN THE TRADITIONAL EXTENDED FAMILY

CULTURAL BACKGROUND INFORMATION

There was order and organization in the traditional family. Nature had an order and organization. This is what the people followed. Each member of the traditional extended family had a role to play in this.

The father was the head of the family. What was to be done was indicated by him. He was the main food gatherer, hunting and bringing in the meat. When he hunted he usually skinned the animal and cut it up for transporting home. If he had young maanikapi apprentices, they would do most of this work, as well as transporting it home. Very little of the animal's parts were discarded.

If he was also the clan leader, the father was the one who decided when a camp was to be taken down and a new one established at a different location. With his wife he led the others in this move. As he matured and gained more experience, he became wiser in his leadership skills.

As a leader, he had a lot of self-respect. As a leader, he knew that he was only one of many leaders of the tribe. The tribe was made up of different clans.

A leader had to earn the respect he got from others. He earned this respect through war, through his acquisitions, bravery, kindness and generosity (he helped others). This is how a man got to be a leader.

The woman was responsible for looking after the immediate home and surroundings. She was responsible for acquiring herbs for medicines. She was also responsible for picking berries, which she would use then and later on throughout the year.

The children were there to help. "This is how our father wanted this done, so that is how we will do it," they said. They all pulled together. That is how there was order.

The elders' role was an advisory one. Great emphasis was placed on their wisdom and knowledge gained through experience. Through this, they were able to caution the ambitious plans of tempestuous youth. From time to time, they also counseled and gave nature lessons to the youth.

The life then was a good life. The people had a happy life. They did not worry. They were independent; they did everything for themselves. They used herbs to cure ailments. They would gather the plants that they used in the spring and summer. They would also prepare the meat after buffalo were killed, for example, in buffalo jump sites. The meat and berries were dried for storage for the winter.

Because it was during the time when men had multiple wives, these women all worked together. Together they sewed new lodges when old ones were becoming too tattered and there were enough skins to put together new ones. All the women of a certain clan would work together.

If one woman found an area which had an abundance of berries, she would alert the other women. All the women and children would congregate at this spot and harvest the bounty.

At night they would study the moon to determine what kind of weather it would be like the following day. "That's the kind of day it's going to be," they would say. Good hunting days were forecast this way. They also used the stars to tell time. The stars of the Big Dipper were used for this. The Evening Star and the Morning Star were also used for telling time.

They followed the day in all the work that they did. They did a lot.

CULTURAL BACKGROUND INFORMATION

The leader advised his wives and the other members of his clan. In preparation for winter, clothing was prepared for the children and the adults. Wood for fuel was gathered and a reliable water source was located.

They also educated themselves. A man instructed young boys on the making of arrows and bows. Then he had them practice using these weapons. He also encouraged them to study nature.

They moved their camps with the ripening of the different berries that they used. They lived healthy lives. Who had glasses? They lived to be 100 years old and their eyes were still healthy. The berries that they ate helped to preserve their teeth.

The people stayed active even in old age. It did not bother the old people to sit on the ground. They could manage the effort of getting up and sitting down without difficulty.

Respect was ingrained into everything that they did. There was very little discord. If one disapproved of the behaviour of certain children, a crier would announce a general message to the effect. Safety from wild animals such as bears, bobcats and cougars was behind this concern.

The people of that time aiksimstatoomiaw opaitapiiwahsowayi, that is, they "thought out their lives." From the bison that their fathers and uncles hunted, the boys made little horses from bones taken from around the hooves of the bison. When someone asked, "Where's the boy?" he would be told, "He is outside, thinking." That is when they "thought out" their future lives.

The same thing happened for girls. When someone asked, "Where are the girls?" she would be told, "They are playing outside, they are thinking." The reason why this play was referred to as "thinking" was that the children were mimicking real life in their play. The boys played with their "horses" and the girls played with their dolls and their "lodges," thinking and planning out their future lives.

Life was good for the people then. There was a spirit of belonging and a sense of family. Everyone worked together. Respect was valued. There was reverence for nature and the spirituality that we were given.

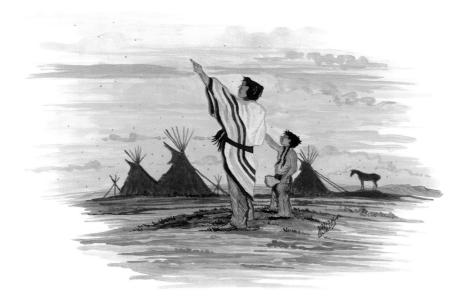

People read the stars to predict weather and to tell time.

ELDER/SURVIVOR G

1964

I was ten or eleven years old when I was placed at the St. Mary's Residential School. The reason I was sent there by my auntie was because she could not afford to look after me. I had been with my auntie because my mother had died. This was in the mid-sixties.

I had some good experiences when I was in residential school. One of these was going out to pray at the grotto. But I also had many bad experiences. I was forced to eat food I did not want. I had to scrub floors. My hair was chopped off without any care for how it would look after.

There was also some physical abuse. If anyone wet their bed, she was whipped without any clothes on by a staff member who also happened to be a brother. This person was very aggressive. We had to do whatever he demanded. We could not talk to one another.

I started to run away from residential school because I felt that I was being treated no better than an animal. I went back to my auntie's place and then my grandparents. I moved around among my aunts' and uncles' places. I also went back to school and finished grade nine in Fort Macleod.

At age sixteen I left home. I was a very independent person and I wanted to look after myself. The choice to leave home was mine alone.

I developed some career goals and I reasoned that I needed a good home to get a good education. I was going to college and then I had a job for one year. I dropped out of school.

I was raped and suffered abuse before I went to Lethbridge. I was sticking around with people I didn't trust and my hopes and dreams were shattered.

After my job experience I realized that I enjoyed working and helping my younger siblings. I went to Edmonton for one year. I had become pregnant. Later, I was in the hospital with a child who was not meant to be. But I kept my baby.

A nurse who worked at the hospital offered me a job to look after her two children. For doing this I had free room and board. I worked as her housekeeper.

Later I moved back home to the reserve and then I moved to Lethbridge. I started to attend college but then I got into a wrong kind of relationship with a man who abused me physically, mentally, verbally and sexually. I went down and I lived in fear. He was so controlling.

I had nowhere to turn but to alcohol. This was not a good place to be. I was made to walk around the house naked. I could not talk to anyone. He also wanted me to give up my child. I also had a son by him.

It took a long time to get over this. Finally he went to jail. I went to Brooks. Alcoholism was stronger than I thought. My children were taken away. I wanted to die. I was just giving up. I ended up in the hospital.

That was my turning point. I surrendered to the Creator. I have been sober now for eleven years. The Creator loves me and he cares for me. I needed to grow spiritually.

The caring part and love is what I have today. I went through struggles. I had to take care.

My ex was interfering in my children. A lot of people were attached to me then. I started to put my foot down. I put a stop to it. I didn't want them to babysit me.

My whole lifestyle is different today. I'm heading in the right direction. With all the qualities I have now, I would like to work. For awhile I took my dad in. I had to look after him and put my life on hold. I'm involved with the Standoff community and I'm involved in AA.

The residential school definitely affected my life. Prior to my going there, my mom and dad had stopped drinking. Even though we had no electricity and no running water, they taught us respect. From them I had picked up a lot of good stuff.

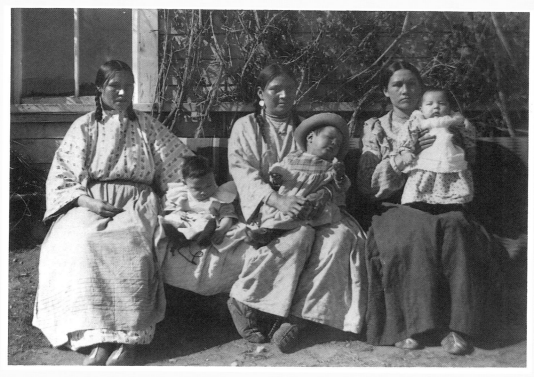

PROVINCIAL ARCHIVES OF ALBERTA/OB.10566

Blood Indian women with children at Standoff, 1935.

ELDER/SURVIVOR H

1954–1965

I attended the St. Paul's Anglican Indian Residential School. The years that I went to school there were 1954 to 1965. I don't really know why I went to school there. All I know is that I was forced into this car which then took me to the school. I don't know if I could have gone to another school.

We were taught reading, math and religion. I did not really get an education but I learned how to work. I learned how to do housework.

I knew only Blackfoot when I went to school. It was the language we used at home. We were not allowed to use Blackfoot at the school. If we were caught speaking it, we would get hit.

There was nothing good about my school experience unless learning how to clean is considered 'good'. The bad things about my school experience were getting hit by supervisors and being forced to do things I didn't want to do.

I don't know about our traditional spirituality or way of praying. I went to residential school so I didn't get to go to or learn about Indian ceremonies. We weren't taught the Indian ways.

There was physical abuse done to me. There was one teacher who wanted you to say "Yes, Miss Higgins" and when I didn't, I would get hit on the ear. As a result, I can't hear out of one ear.

My sister could not drink milk. It made her very sick. We had porridge every morning and she would eat it without milk. Somehow one of the teachers found out about this and one day put milk in her cereal and told her to eat it. Because my table was done, we had left the cafeteria. One of other kids came running out to get me and told me that the teacher was beating up my sister. I went back in and I saw the teacher forcing my sister to eat the cereal with milk. She forced the food down her throat. There was blood all over her face because the skin on the sides of her mouth had been torn by the force-feeding. We ran away later.

There were three men, the teachers and supervisor who abused girls. The principal forced me to go up north to supervise at another school. At that school I was told that I could hit or slap the girls if they didn't do things 'right'. As a supervisor I was told that I could beat up the students. One of the teachers who transferred from St. Paul's said that I had to go out with him. I was scared of getting into trouble so I did. He would pick me up and take me to the show. He was going to the hospital for surgery and said that I had to come and visit him or he would think that I was running around with someone else. He told me to live with him. I didn't want to so I made excuses to put him off. Then one of the other staff, an Eskimo girl, told me that I didn't have to do what he said. I was a staff member now, not a student. She told me to go to him the next day and tell him this. She said she would go with me and she did. I told him and said that when I got back to the reserve I was going to tell on him. He was very upset and told me that I could get anyone I wanted to come up and join me. I told him who I wanted to come and work with me. This person joined me soon after. The teacher never bothered me after that time. I do know that at the school the male teachers and supervisors would force the girls to go to their rooms with them. Everyone knew what they were doing to the girls.

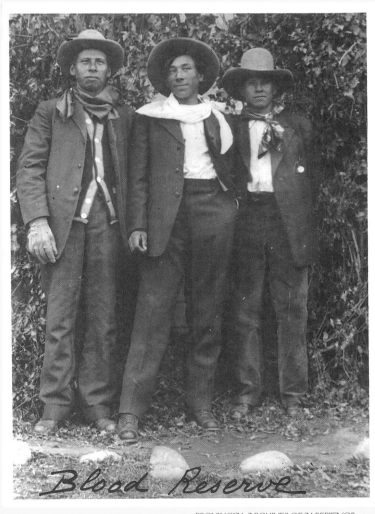

Blood Reserve

PROVINCIAL ARCHIVES OF ALBERTA/OB.9044

Young Men at Blood Reserve, Standoff.

ELDER/SURVIVOR I

1953

When I was six years old I went to the St. Mary's Indian Residential School. At the time, I didn't understand why I was being sent away. My feelings were that my mom did not want me around. I did not even know that the reason my older siblings were gone all the time was that they were in residential school. I just knew they were leaving all the time.

I enjoyed the school part of residential school. I didn't mind learning but I didn't enjoy living in residential school. When I started learning it made a big difference, even though I could not understand why I had to live away from home.

I spoke fluent Blackfoot when I went to school. Because of this I went through hell with the nuns because they wanted us to speak English. I made two very good friends. The three of us used to talk secretly to each other in Blackfoot. When some older girls told on us we got slapped on the head or we were hit on the head with bells. There was no one there I could look to for help because my older sisters were in different playrooms.

However, the three of us decided we would stick together and whenever an older girl told on us, we would get even with her later on. When this happened we would wait for her on the stairs and when she came by alone, we would jump her and beat her up.

There was one nun whom we could not understand when she tried to speak English. We just could not understand her. Yet we were expected to speak English.

I had nobody to turn to except my two friends. After we got picked on too many times, we got rebellious and fought back. When I got a little older, I started taking off from home when it was time to return to the residential school. I didn't want to go back.

When my grandma died, the priest would not let us go home for the weekend because he knew we would go to her funeral. He did not want us to go because our grandmother was Anglican. We were kept at the school. We were not allowed to mourn her. All we could do was look out the dorm windows from the top floor and see the funeral procession from a distance. Because of this, my grandmother's death was not a reality. I did not accept that she was dead. She had only gone somewhere. When I asked my mother later where grandma was, she did not say anything to me.

I really blame the government because we were not taught what we needed to know about love. No one really cared about us; the nuns just watched us. We were there only to be told what to do. We were not taught to love or to care about people.

I tried to like the nuns but I couldn't. There was only one who was really good to me. She favoured me, I think because I was smart in class.

I never experienced any sexual abuse but I did experience physical and emotional abuse. In spite of my experiences in residential school, I still have faith in the church. I ask God to help me.

Today I check out everyone first. It's the people who did the harm to me. I was a tomboy in school and everybody was my friend. By the time I was in intermediate girls, I was blamed for any little thing that went wrong. If I had any privileges, they were taken away on a nun's whim.

I was not perfect. I did things I was not supposed to do but I did them for a reason. When I got into my teens, I told myself I was never going to allow the nuns or priests to make me cry. They never did.

One day in class, I noticed a blood stain on another girl's dress. She sat in a row in front of me. She did not realize that she was having a period. After I told her about it, she asked me to walk behind her, to go to the office. She wanted to get permission to go to the residence to change. When we got to the office there was no one there.

We decided we would quickly run to the other building so that she could change into clean clothes. We did. Later on this girl was called to the principal's office. When she came back she was crying. She held her hands out to show me that she had been strapped there. They looked red and puffy. She told me that the principal wanted to see me too.

When I got to the principal's office, I tried to explain why we had done what we did. He insisted that I should not have accompanied the other girl so that no one could see the embarrassing blood stain.

Without hearing me, he pulled out his thick heavy strap and ordered me to hold out my hand. He held his right arm far back behind him. I think he did this to get more momentum when he strapped me. Just when the strap was going to connect with my hand. I quickly moved it. He hit himself in the crotch! This happened two more times. Finally he ordered me to kneel on the floor by the couch. He was going to strap my 'behind'. Fortunately for me, I had on one of those crinoline skirts, which flared out. Every time he strapped me and connected with my body, my clothing protected me. I pretended to be really hurting and loudly cried out mock sobs.

He eventually stopped and before I left he told me to shut the door behind me. As I was shutting the door I stuck out my tongue at him and yelled "*Yahai* Father, you didn't hurt me!" After that he did not like me, even when I became an adult. He got back his own medicine.

When my mother brought us food at the residence, the nuns would take some and give it to their pets. They lied to us in a lot of ways. If we lied to them they beat us up. I don't blame all the priests and nuns, just the bad ones. Why did they do bad things to us to make us feel bad? They're supposed to show love and kindness. They wanted us to respect them but they did not respect us.

Us Indians were put through a lot. If things had been different for me in how they treated me, I might have graduated from grade 12.

We went to mass every morning. We used to have to stand a lot. Some of the weaker students would faint. We were not even allowed to help them when they fell!

I think that my experience at residential school affected every relationship I ever had. When things got rough, I shipped out like I did when I ran away from residential school. Now I am finally changing.

No one ever listened to me in residential school. None of the adults there ever took the time to find out how we were. I find it hard to forgive them. If there were residential schools today, I would never send my kids there.

Some experiences were very humiliating and destructive. One of these times was when I saw a girl get strapped in front of all of us. They pulled up her dress and the principal strapped her in front of all the junior girls!

We could not look out the windows. We were forbidden to do so many things. It was just like a prison. But I did enjoy going to classes because we had fun in there.

I have not joined in the lawsuit being brought against the people who ran the residential schools. Some of the people suing never suffered like some others did. I don't want people to dislike nuns and priests. I just think that they sent us all the bad ones.

The food was awful—burnt porridge, not enough to eat. Yet when we passed by the priests' dining room, we saw all the good food laid out. No wonder some kids stole food! It was even a treat to get an apple or an orange. And if we didn't want to eat some food, we were forced to eat it anyway.

I'm a little wary of priests and nuns now. They could have used their common sense.

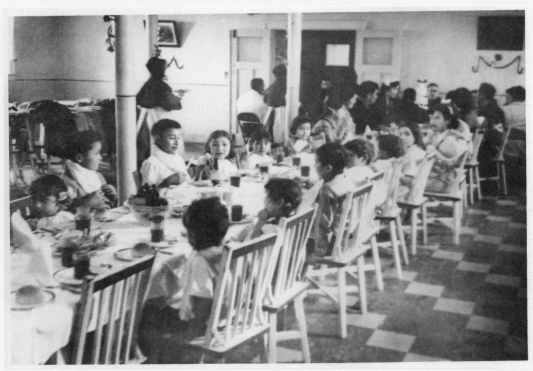

Mealtime for residential students. (Nuns-Cardston)

ELDER/SURVIVOR J

I went to the St. Paul's Anglican Indian Residential School in the 1960s. An older brother and sister were there already. We had transportation problems. That's why we attended that school. I guess I could have gone to Cardston.

1960s

We were taught play activities, social skills, learning manners and basic education stuff. This was useful to me later on after I left school.

Blackfoot was my language when I went to school. It was the language we used at home. At the school we were not allowed to speak Blackfoot. I was once hit by a teacher for saying my Blackfoot name.

I learned independence when I went to school. This has helped me now as a parent. I would never want my children to go through what some of the kids had to endure at residential school. If I was a teacher, I would never treat my students the way we were treated there.

I believe that our traditional spirituality/Indian religion is the best for me. I do not attend the Anglican church anymore.

The kind of abuse that I suffered in school was the bullying by other students. I was a teacher's pet and, because of this, one girl threw me off the swings. This was one time. Another was when this same bully pushed me down the stairs because she was jealous of the teacher's attention to me.

I saw other students being abused. One time when I was a junior, the boys and girls were all going downstairs. On the way down we witnessed a boy being strapped with his pants off. There were a lot of incidents like this.

Residential school was a lonely place for a lot of the students. We had no choice but to be placed there. Bullying made it a pitiful experience for many of the students.

ADAM DELANY

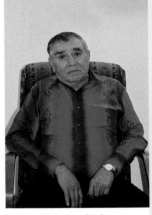

Mamio'kakiikin (Adam Delaney), Kainai elder and grandfather to the Iitskinayiiksi.

I do not profess to know everything but I will give as much information as I can about the past. I was given this information by my grandfathers and grandmothers.

Before naapiikoaksi arrived we did everything for ourselves. We governed ourselves on this land which I will call an island.

The Creator put us on this land where the mountains are, where the prairie begins and where Mookowansin is located. This is where the Siksikai'tsitapi were put.

Even though we lived here, we knew much of what was located to the south (pihkoohtsi-aamskaapoohtsi [now]) and in all other directions. Our people travelled and some even went as far as the ocean. Our ancestors met the other tribes, which were also put here on this island. There were many other tribes put on this island.

GENDER ROLES

In the past there were definite roles for the man and the woman. The man was a man and the woman was a woman.

The man took care of everything which his wife and children needed to survive. He travelled long distances to do what he had to do.

The woman, on the other hand, took care of her children. She raised her children and looked after the household. She kept things organized in her home.

If a man had a son he taught him how to hunt. He taught him also the art of war. This was in the days before the gun was brought in. He did not have too much to say about how a daughter was raised.

If, however, he noticed something about a daughter's behaviour which he did not like, he talked to his wife about it and expected that the right thing would be done. "You look after it," he would tell his wife.

If there was no improvement after the woman had reprimanded her daughter, a grandmother was asked to intervene. (It is sometimes a wonder how a child will not listen to her parents, but she will listen to her grandparents.)

The same thing was done for boys. If a son would not listen to his father, the father would ask a grandfather to talk to the son.

That is how we were raised in the past. We were counselled about everything. That is why we had an orderly society. Whenever a person did not heed advice and he continued to go against the counselling of his elders, his behaviour was noted. He gained notoriety. "Such and such is like this," the people said. But it should be noted that the people who followed order and the good life were in a majority.

SPIRITUALITY

From this, let us go to prayer. More of our people prayed in the past. They prayed to Ihtsipaitapiiyio'pa and to Naato'si the sun. In their prayers they included the water, the mountains and the earth. All the birds and land animals were also mentioned. What was used for smudging was also included. Everything that was in our prayers was evident.

Paramount in our prayers was the search for harmony in our relationships with others. Not to be able to get along with others was considered very bad.

We had our songs and we had our holy food.

AFTER CONTACT WITH NAAPIIKOAIKSI:

There was a lot of disruption caused to our society after Naapiikoaiksi arrived here.

First of all, they settled on our land, wherever they fancied building a house. That is why we had to fight them. Many of our people received their names because they took rifles away from them.

They moved our society in a bad way. Our people were strong. That is why we are still here. Naapiikoana realized this. They realized that our spirituality made us strong. That is why they decided to make treaty with us. They began this process in the east and they made their way westward.

By the time they got here, it was up to treaty number seven. After we signed the treaty and we had agreed to live in peace, Naapiikoana went too far and took away our livelihood. They were greedy.

Then they began to educate our people according to their way. Our people suffered a lot at that time. Some of the rations, which our people were given, were laced with poison. Some of the blankets, which they gave us, were infected with diseases against which we had no immunity. Many of our ceremonial tools were taken from us and now these are scattered in far off lands.

Some say that our people sold these. No, they were not sold. After we had signed the treaty and agreed that we would not fight anymore, Naapiikoaiksi took advantage of this. Whatever means we had to maintain an orderly society they tried to take away, and they did at every opportunity. That is why I say that we did not sell our sacred objects. We almost lost everything. We almost lost.

Our grandfathers did not speak naapiikoai'powahsini and they could not read it. As a consequence of this, they were mislead. They made some decisions based on misconceptions. After all of this, our people began to be educated according to their way.

We were a stubborn people. That is why we are still here.

Our education according to the ways of another society began. Learning to fear our traditional ways was included in this education. Gradually, we were brainwashed into believing that our ways were wrong, that they were evil and that they were to be avoided at all cost.

We come to today, to the present. Sometimes when I try to talk to my grandchildren and other young people, they tell me that our traditional ways belong to the past, to another time. No, that is not true. Our way of life, our spirituality will never stop.

It has happened on more than one occasion that individual members of our tribe will go a long way in becoming educated according to the ways of the outside. Sometime later, these same members turn around and embrace our spirituality. This tells me that our ways are not of the past.

If we trace our lives back, we will not find Naapiikoaiksi on this island. If you trace your life back through the generations, you will discover only your grandfathers and grandmothers. They are the ones who put you here.

OUR LEADERSHIP

When we chose our leaders in the past, we always chose those who lived well-ordered lives. We did not refer to such a person as "chief," we just said that this person "led us" and that we "followed this person."

Red Crow was our leader when Treaty 7 was signed. He signed the treaty for us. Naapiikoaiksi have made comments that he was greedy and that is why he made some of the decisions that he made. He was not. It is their greed that makes them say this.

The designation of "chief" was formalized and the twelve councillors we call Maohkotooksskaiksi was established after kinniinaysini was introduced by the government.

Voting as we have it today was another new practice established to choose our leaders. Prior to this, the process was not so formal. A leader was simply chosen by how he lived his life. There was evidence that a person selected as leader lived an orderly life and that he was a compassionate person.

There was no such thing as "If you vote for me I will do this." A person did not need to boast about what he was going to do if he was selected. The process was very different.

Now that we have learned to read and write English, we have confused our lifestyle with that of naapiikoaiksi. Many a niitsitapiikaon will use naapiipaitapiiwahsini until he comes to a tough situation. Then where does he fall back on? He goes back to Niitsitapiipaitapiiwahsini.

The reason I am saying these things is to talk about them so that we think about them. Today, many of our young people do not listen to us. They can even charge us if we try to correct them physically.

CHILD-REARING

In the past, a mother and father talked to their children. If a child was not behaving according to the accepted ways, the parents talked to him. If that did not work, the grandparents were called in to help. Usually this was the extent of the problem. However, in case this did not work, then an extreme measure was employed.

Aisski'tstaiksi were used then. These were people whose role was to frighten children when they were not listening to their parents. Because they were frightening, children almost always changed their behaviour for the better.

Parents invited aisski'tstaiksi to their homes when the need arose. A person who was used as a "child frightener" knew when his services were required. Usually a child's reputation preceded him. It usually only took one scary visit and the problem was solved. Parents only had to mention inviting a frightener again and the child settled down again.

We helped each other in many ways. This was only one way. Today, if we asked someone to serve as a frightener, some parents would probably misunderstand his purpose and get after the person instead.

THE NEED FOR EDUCATION TODAY

The reason I am talking this way is to emphasize the fact that we need education today. I myself have a very poor education background and I know how important education is today.

We are coming to the point now that we will be running everything for ourselves, that is if we do not allow ourselves to be overcome by outsiders and we keep our land.

Every year, the curriculum keeps changing and students need to learn more and more. This is why it is important to complete our education. Computers and technology make it seem as if we will never learn enough. But we cannot give up.

One thing that beats us is the clock. Many of our people are achieving a good education. However, we are not used to doing things on time. Our concept of time is different.

Another thing which we are not used to yet is how to manage money. There are some people who have made good money in the past but they have returned to the street corner without a penny in their pockets.

According to our traditional way, the rationale for doing something is because it will help our people. If it will not help our people, we will not do it. This is different from the naapiikoaiksi, where their aim for doing something is very personal. They will do something and complete it because they are doing it only for themselves.

Our society is different. What we strive for, we strive for not only for ourselves but for our people as well. But there are some of us who are beginning to follow naapiipaitapiiwahsini.

For myself, I could be very well off today if I had had a good education in the past. Now that I am seventy years old, I think back on it. My inability to follow the clock and to save money caused some of this. I made good money but I wasted it on having a good time.

I worked with many different kinds of people and I made a good living. But I accepted a lot of the outside vices and my life for a long time was not a good one. When I was fairly old, I made the decision to turn my life around and examine the teachings of my grandparents, and what my mother and father had taught me. I discovered that these were good and that they were made for us. We were given this way of life and it is good.

Now that I am getting old, I am being asked to serve as a grandfather and counsellor in many different things. Whenever I consider matters, I always realize how lucky we are that we were given the things that we have.

As I have already stated, we chose our leaders in the past based on the good that they had done and were continuing to do. Now I fear that we are choosing some shady people. We vote for these people for selfish reasons. We believe that they can do something personal for us. We are also voting for some people because they are related to us. These are wrong reasons for choosing a leader.

Our way is different from this. We always think of the collective good because our land belongs to all of us.

We are becoming too influenced by the ways of the outside. It is only because we are stubborn that we are able to maintain some of our traditional ways.

Teachers have a very important function in the present time. They are like the parents today. The days are gone when parents were able to stay at home and raise their children. Today many parents work and sometimes children leave an empty house when they go off to school.

The teachers are the ones who advise these children on what is right and wrong. Many times it happens that parents go somewhere in the evenings after school. Children are left again without anybody to talk to them. Sometimes another adult is thwarted in counselling children when they do something wrong because he/she knows that the parents will not like it.

By the time some parents realize how much counselling their children need, it is too late. They are in trouble or they are drinking alcohol or smoking some drug. This is what naapiipaitapiiwahsini has done to us.

Our traditional way was to counsel a child from when he or she was very young. A child was always counselled so that he/she contributed to the well-being of the tribe. A child who did not follow this order was considered notorious.

At the present time it seems that there are more young people who follow naapiipaitapiiwahsini. Fewer of our young people follow the old way.

I have lived according to both ways; I have done both ways. I think my life today would have been better if I had returned to the traditional life sooner.

I know that we cannot escape naapia'pii. We need education in order to live in today's world. Get all the education you can. But leave out the bad part, the part that will hurt you. Look to your native spirituality for strength. That is our greatest strength.

Whenever we can make a choice between our traditional way and naapia'pii, we should always follow the traditional way. It is real and genuine.

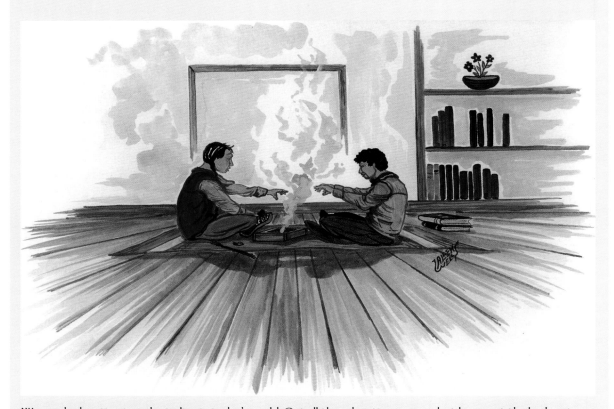

We need education in order to live in today's world. Get all the education you can but leave out the bad part, the part that will hurt you. Look to your native spirituality for strength.

GOAL(S)	OBJECTIVE(S)	CULTURAL CONCEPT
1. To realize that there were two industrial schools in southern Alberta. 2. To understand why these schools did not last very long.	1. Students will discuss the curriculum of these schools. 2. Students will explain why many parents would not send their children to industrial schools. 3. Students will be able to make inferences from information given.	In the last two decades of the nineteenth century, two industrial schools were established in southern Alberta to help acculturate Treaty 7 tribes.

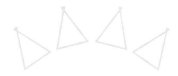

STUDENT ACTIVITIES	EVALUATION ACTIVITIES	RESOURCES
1. Students will read/listen to cultural background information. 2. Students will complete a chart, as illustrated, using the information about the sixty students from St. Joseph's Industrial School. 3. Students will find and interview the descendents of Blood Indians who attended industrial schools and develop a biography of at least one of these former students.	1. Students will design a quiz on Indian industrial schools. 2. Student-designed quiz will be given. 3. Class will discuss industrial schools.	1. *Kitomahkitapiiminnooniksi—Stories from Our Elders*, Vol. 1–3 2. *My People the Bloods*, Mike Mountain Horse 3. Elders from list 4. Descendents of industrial school graduates

CULTURAL BACKGROUND INFORMATION

Toward the latter part of the nineteenth century, two residential "industrial" schools were established by the federal government in southern Alberta. Under the direction of Father Lacombe and the Oblate Fathers of Mary Immaculate, the St. Joseph's Industrial School was established in 1886. This was the Roman Catholic School. It was also known as "Dunbow." The Calgary Indian Industrial School, was established later, in the 1890s, and was under the Church of England.

The philosophy for the establishment of these schools was to remove the Indian child from his community and his home so that traditional influences were also removed. The curriculum of these schools was geared mostly to produce students who could farm, do carpentry work and be good general labourers. The girls were taught housewife duties and housework so that they could become good homemakers. Most students also learned reading, writing and mathematics skills in the half-day of instruction they received daily. Of course, they were also given religious instruction.

Attendance at these schools was not good. School and government officials could not induce many students from the Treaty 7 tribes to attend their institutions. Especially in the light of so many students acquiring tuberculosis, many parents would not part with their children.

Many of the graduates of these schools became successful farmers and ranchers. James Gladstone was one of these graduates. He attended the Calgary Industrial School. So did Willy Scraping White, who later became a much revered elder among Kainai. Another was Maurice Many Fingers, who attended Dunbow. Frank Red Crow, the adopted son of Mi'kiai'sto (Red Crow), also attended Dunbow. Tom Three Persons of Calgary Stampede fame graduated from Dunbow in 1906. He was also a very successful rancher.

By the turn of the century, the Anglicans and the Roman Catholics also had mission boarding schools on the Blood Reserve. It was more economical for the government to fund these new schools. Not only were they more accessible to students, but they could also achieve the same purpose as the industrial schools. By the second decade of the twentieth century, these schools were firmly entrenched in Niitsitapi life on the Blood Reserve.

The following pages contain information from the "Register of Admissions" for St. Joseph's Industrial School.

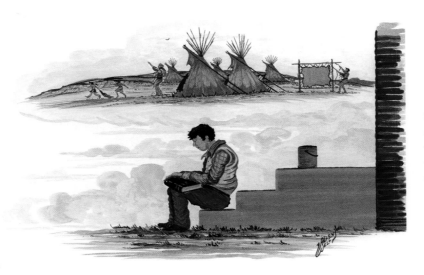

Students were removed not only from their families but also from their language and culture.

ST. JOSEPH'S INDUSTRIAL SCHOOL, DAVIDSBURG, 1886–1922
REGISTRE DES ADMISSIONS, #1–370
(COMMONLY REFERRED TO AS "DUNBOW")

W.D. Davis	Was nine years old when he was discharged on 27th of April, 1890. Period in the school was 34 days. He was at Standard I. His father the "Critter" claimed his boy back, all efforts to oppose him were in vain.
Johnny Blood	Was nine years old at discharge on 28th of September, 1891. Period in school was two years, 11 months and 28 days. State of education on discharge was Standard I. "When he came to school, had a sore knee; shortly after had his leg amputated, and was thus unable to attend class. At the end of September 1891, he died from bleeding of the lungs."
#86 Alfred Young	Was 14 years old when he was discharged on 26th of August 1893. Period in the school was 4 years and 5 months. He was Standard II on discharge. His trade was "Fatigue." "He was a very good boy, and always very willing at work. Employed at ordinary fatigue work. He died after only day's illness from excessive eating of chokecherries."
#157 Jas. Fox	Aged 17 years old when discharged on 21st of February 1897. His period in the school was 2 years, 8 months, 21 days. He was discharged at Standard II level. His trade was Farmer—all branches—fair worker and obedient. Died on Blood Reserve, February 21, 1897, was absent from the school on two occasions on sick leave—was consumptive and physically weak. Died on reserve.
#13 Alex Stevens	Age 20 at discharge on 23 June, 1897. His period in school was 7 years, 1 month, 6 days. He was at Standard II. He was a "Carpenter - good progress works well." "Has been absent from the school for over 2 years previous to his discharge. Worked at his trade on the Blood Reserve."
#143 Joe Aberdeen	[probably aged 18 years old on discharge] This took place on 23 June 1897. His period in school was 2 years, 7 months, 3 days. He was at Standard II. His trade or industry taught and proficiency in it was "farmer—a very good worker… Discharged to begin life on his own account—Took up a place on the reserve and is married."
#155 Hugh Brewer	Age 19 at discharge, which was October 12, 1897. His period in school was 3 years, 5 months, 7 days. He was at Standard I. His trade was "Farming—a very good worker… Can speak English and this is about all—was too old when admitted but is a very good worker." (A later entry indicated that he "died at Stony Mountain Penitentiary.")

#144 Jack Crow	Age 20 at discharge on July 16, 1898. His period in school was 4 years, 4 months, 25 days. He was a Standard I. His trade was "farmer—good and strong worker… "Too old when admitted to learn much in school room. Returned to the Bloods. Married and keeps cattle. Died on reserve."
#146 Harry Wells	Age 18 at discharge on July 16, 1898. His period in school was 4 years 4 months 25 days. He was a Standard II. "Farmer—fairly proficient… Returned to the Blood Reserve, died since from consumption."
#156 Stephen Fox	18 years old at discharge on July 16, 1898. His period in school was 4 years, 2 months, 4 days. He was at Standard II (well advanced). Farmer and Carpenter. "Did very well while in school. Keeps very tidy on the reserve; has cattle."
#170 Duncan Shade	8 years old at discharge on July 16, 1898. His period in school was 1 year, 10 months, 27 days. He was at Standard I. He could speak some English. Farmer fair worker. "Not bright, but of good dispositions, died on Blood Reserve 1907."
#165 George Vielle	18 years old at discharge on July 8, 1899. His period in school was 4 years, 10 months, 8 days. He was at Standard II (on admission) and Standard IV on discharge. Carpentering and farming, a little of each. "Intelligent boy; returned to the Bloods."
#166 Frank Red Crow	17 years old at discharge on July 8, 1899. His period in school was 4 years, 6 months, 8 days. He was Standard I on admission and Standard IV on discharge. Carpenter—good and intelligent worker. "Returned to his guardian 'Red Crow' of the Bloods."
#171 Percy Steele	19 years old at discharge on July 8, 1899. His period in school was 4 years, 3 months, 17 days. He was Standard II on discharge. Farmer—good and strong worker. "Came back to the school in May 1900, and married pupil Eliza Montcalm. Died on Blood Reserve, 1906."

CULTURAL BACKGROUND INFORMATION

"The following three pupils were discharged, by order of Mr. Laird, because their stepfather 'Heavy Head' was married in the Protestant Church and these children were to follow that religion."

#149 Jos. Trollinger

13 years old on discharge on April 17, 1900.
Time at school was 6 years, 1 month, 26 days. He was at Standard I. "Fatigue—very dull no proficiency—could talk English."

#31 Minnie Trollinger

(Doherty) 15 years old on discharge on April 7, 1900.
Time at school was 8 years, 11 months. She was at Standard III. "Housework—fair progress."

#043 Katie Trollinger

17 years old on discharge on April 7, 1900.
Time at school was 6 years, 1 month, 26 days. She was at Standard II—had "impediment in the speech."
"Housework—better at work than in class."

#90 Paul Fox

20 years of age at discharge on May 22, 1900.
Time at school was 10 years, 9 months, 22 days. At Standard V on discharge. "Very good progress. Carpenter—not strong… Went to the Blood Reserve where he secured work at his trade."

#044 Emma Fox

16 years old at discharge on July 10, 1900.
Time at school was 6 years, 4 months, 12 days. Was at Standard I at entrance and Standard III by discharge. Housework—good. "Married No.53, John English."

#177 Jas. Wells

18 years old at discharge on July 3, 1901.
Time at school was 3 years, 10 months, 15 days. Was at Standard II. Farming—"fair… Had reached age limit."

#030 Lilly Mills

17 years old at discharge on May 4, 1901.
Time at school was 9 years, 11 months, 16 days. Was at Standard IV Housework. "Allowed home to get married."

#048 Annie English

18 years old at discharge on July 16, 1901.
Time at school was 7 years, 1 month, 9 days. At Standard IV. Housework. "Had reached age limit."

#169 Peter Sleeps on Top

14 years old at discharge on May 02, 1903.
Time at school was 7 years, 6 months. At Standard II. Fatigue—good. "Allowed home on sick leave, 17 May, 1902 died."

#111 Michael Blood — 18 years old at discharge on July 28, 1903. Time at the school was 12 years, 2 months, 10 days. At Standard III. Farming—"fair... Had reached age limit."

#138 Jos. Beebe — 18 years old at discharge on July 7, 1903. Time at school was 9 years, 9 months, 7 days. At Standard V. Farming—"very good... Had reached age limit."

#135 Henry Mills — 18 years old at discharge on July 10, 1905. Time at school was 11 years, 7 months, 21 days. At Standard V. Farming—"good... Had reached age limit."

#159 Nick King — 19 years old at discharge on July 10, 1905. Time at school was 5 years, 2 months, 5 days. Began at Standard I and finished at Standard III. Farming—"good... Had reached age limit."

#212 Frank Wolf Child — 18 years old at discharge on July 10, 1905. Time at school was 4 years, 1 month, 21 days. Started at Standard I and finished at Standard II. Carpentry—"g... Had reached age limit."

#167 Joe Devine — 19 years old at discharge on July 11, 1906. Time at school was 11 years, 7 months, 24 days. Completed Standard VI. Farming—"g... Had reached age limit."

#172 Walter Singer — 18 years old at discharge on July 11, 1906. Time at school was 11 years, 3 months, 2 days. At Standard II. Farming—"fair... Had reached age limit."

#192 Peter Bear — 16 years old at discharge on July 11, 1906. Time at school was 9 years, 1 month, 2 days. At Standard II. Farming—"fair... Discharged by authority of Indian Commissioner."

#226 Thos Three Persons — 18 years old at discharge on July 11, 1906. Time at school was 3 years, 2 months, 6 days Left at Standard II. Farming—"g... Had reached age limit."

#046 Eliza Frank

18 years old at discharge on July 26, 1906.
Time at school was 12 years, 2 months. At Standard V.
Housewifery duties—"good… Had reached age limit."

#227 Thos. Russel

17 years old at discharge on June 02, 1907.
Time at the school was 3 years, 11 months, 3 days. Went
from Standard II to Standard III. Farming—"good…
Discharged by authority of the Commissioner to go home in
order to assist his blind father."

#140 Emile Scout

18 years old at discharge on July 03, 1907.
Time at school was 13 years, 9 months, 1 day. At Standard
VI. Farming—"g… Had reached age limit."

#231 Maurice ManyFingers

18 years at discharge on July 03, 1907.
Time at school was 3 years. Went from Standard I to
Standard III. Farming—"g… Had reached age limit."

#224 Thos Many Feathers

18 years at discharge on August 02, 1907.
Time at school was 4 years. Went to Standard III.
Farming—"g… Had reached age limit."

#154 Chas. Blood

18 years old at discharge on July 06, 1908.
Time at school was 14 years, 1 month, 24 days. At Standard
V. Farming—"v.g.… Age limit."

#054 Agnes King

18 years old at discharge on March05, 1908.
Time at school was 12 years, 10 months, 24 days. At
Standard IV. Housewifery duties—"v.g.… Discharged to
marry graduate (213) Peter Single Rider, Blood Reservation."

#232 Thos. Eagle Child

18 years old at discharge on July 10/1909
Time at school was 5 years, 1 month. At Standard V.
Farmer—"good… Had reached age limit."

#083 Annie Pace

18 years old at discharge on December 10, 1910.
Time at the school was 2 years, 7 months, 10 days. Began at
Standard IV and left at Standard VI. Housework and
sewing—"g… Age limit."

CULTURAL BACKGROUND INFORMATION

#239 Henry Blackwater

18 years old at discharge on August 20, 1910. Time at school was 5 years 3 months 18 days. Began at Standard II and went as far as Standard V. Farming—"good... Age limit."

#240 Dave Mills

18 years old at discharge in July 1911.
Time at school was 6 years, 2 months. Went from Standard II to Standard VI. "Farmer" "Age limit—living on Blood Reserve."

#267 Harry Big Throat

18 years old at discharge on June 30, 1911.
Time at the school was 2 years, 2 months. Went from Standard IV to Standard VI. Farming—"v.g.... Age limit."

#268 Aloy Many Fingers

18 years old at discharge on June 30, 1911
Time at school was 2 years, 2 months. Went from Standard 3 to Standard 5. Farming—"good... Age limit."

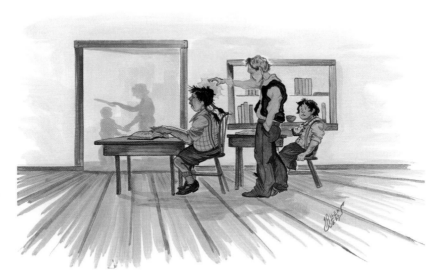

Some students were physically abused because they were unable to understand concepts they were studying.

GREAT GRANDMOTHER'S RESIDENTIAL SCHOOL EXPERIENCE—1926

GOAL(S)

1. To understand that the Indian residential school (I.R.S.) of the 1920s did not concentrate on academic education.
2. To understand that the I.R.S. of the 1920s was regimented and restrictive.

OBJECTIVE(S)

1. Students will discuss the education process of the I.R.S. in the 1920s.
2. Students will discuss how I.R.S. students were sometimes abused by school personnel in order to "break" them in.
3. Students will recall and explain the traditional process of counselling; how young people were counselled and how the I.R.S. interfered in this process.
4. Students will discuss how the use of "modelling" was interfered with by the I.R.S.

CULTURAL CONCEPT

The I.R.S. interfered with traditional practices such as child counselling and child welfare.

RESOURCES

1. *Kitomahkitapiiminnooniksi— Stories from Our Elders*, Vol. 1–3
2. Herbert First Rider, Elsie First Rider, Harold Healy, Jean Healy, Mary Singer, Isabel Spear Chief, Jennie Neilson, Wallace Oka, Irene Day Rider, Bernard Tall Man, Rita Tall Man, Tom White Man, Rachel Crying Head, Flora Zaharia, Laura Madl, Mary Pace, Pete Standing Alone, Rosie Yellow Feet, Bernard Plain Woman, Rita Frank, Mary First Rider, Angeline Standing Alone, Ralph Bottle, Irene Small Eyes, Lucy Black Plume, Alvine Crop Eared Wolf, Rita Calf Robe, Louise Brave Rock, Donald Black Plume, Mervin Brave Rock, Irene Tail Feathers, Josephine Melting Tallow, Eva Hind Bull, Annie Heavy Head, Pauline Dempsey, Chester Bruised Head, Leona Eagle Speaker, Mary Louise Oka, Mary Stella Bare Shin Bone, Florence Red Crow.

STUDENT ACTIVITIES

1. Students will read/listen to cultural background information.
2. In cooperative groups of four, students will list student activities in the I.R.S. and the positive and negative aspects about each.
3. Invite elders who were formerly I.R.S. students to discuss the traditional counselling practice(s) and how orphaned children were adopted and raised by relatives.

EVALUATION ACTIVITIES

1. Cooperative groups of four will generate a quiz on I.R.S. activities to teach students.
2. In cooperative groups of four, students will choose an elder born in the 1920s or 1930s and complete a "models" poster of that elder. One or more members will personally interview this elder.

CULTURAL BACKGROUND INFORMATION

See Lesson 12 Tsiinaakii (Mrs. Rosie Red Crow) "Great Grandmother's Residential School Experience" interview section.

GOAL(S)

1. To understand that the Indian residential school (I.R.S.), isolated young Kainai members not only from their tribe but from the larger Canadian society.
2. To understand that parents had no choice or very limited choice of where their children would be educated.
3. To understand that one of the aims of the government in establishing the I.R.S. was to extinguish Kainai language and culture.

OBJECTIVE(S)

1. Students will discuss the "registration process" of Indian residential schools.
2. Students will describe the curriculum of I.R.S. and what it prepared the I.R.S. graduate for.
3. Students will describe the effects of the poor diet at the I.R.S.
4. Students will describe the theology of Niitsitapiaatsimoihkaani and compare and contrast it with Christianity.

CULTURAL CONCEPT

The Indian residential schools on the Blood Reserve were not an extension of the Kainai home. In fact, these schools attempted to do away with Kainai language and culture.

STUDENT ACTIVITIES

1. Take the class on a walking tour of R.C.C.C and tell students that this used to be St. Mary's R.C. I.R.S.
2. Have the students draw a diagram of each floor while listening to guides describing the school as it used to be.
3. Have students draw a layout of the old St. Mary's I.R.S. (exterior), as described by guide.
4. With the students, read elder/survivor stories AA and BB.
5. Students will prepare questions for elders.
6. Students will listen to two elders recount their experiences when they went to school at St. Mary's I.R.S.
7. Students will read the "spirituality" section and ask elders about spirituality.

EVALUATION ACTIVITIES

1. In cooperative groups of four, students will prepare a quiz. These questions will include the curriculum of the I.R.S. and the outcome, cultural differences of school and home.
2. In these same groups students will prepare a short, two-page report comparing and contrasting an I.R.S. with schools today or compare and contrast Kainai society of 1930s with Kainai society today, or compare and contrast Niitsitapiaatsimoihkaani with Christianity.

RESOURCES

1. *Kitomahkitapiiminnooniksi— Stories from Our Elders*, Vol. 1–3.
2. Mrs. Irene Day Rider, Mrs. Rachel Crying Head

CULTURAL BACKGROUND INFORMATION

See Residential School interview—Elder/Survivor K and Elder/Survivor L.

ELDER/SURVIVOR K

1937

We were living in Lethbridge and that is where Naatoyiikakato'si came to pick me up. I went to St. Mary's Indian Residential School. There were three of us who were picked up in Lethbridge.

When we arrived at the school it was night. We were sent to bed. In the morning, after we got up, we had our hair cut short. Some of the older girls had told us earlier that this would happen. They also told us that our own clothes would be put away. We would not see them again until the following June, just before we left for summer holidays.

In spite of the warning, we cried when our hair was cut. We did not really understand what was happening. I really depended on this one girl who knew her way around. She seemed to know what the nuns were doing all the time. In the morning I worked. In the afternoon was when I went to classes.

I worked in the laundry. I cleaned and washed the stairs. There were quite a few of us who worked and only went to school for half-a-day.

I had been in school for about two years when I suffered an injury to one of my eyes. I was not brought to the hospital but was sent up to bed in the dormitory. Later I was brought to the hospital.

My mother heard that I was in the hospital. They were camping close to the hospital because my father was helping with the construction of the Roxy Theatre in Cardston. My mother and I were still visiting when I saw that Naatoyiikakato'si had come to the hospital to pick me up.

"Here comes Naatoyiikakato'si to bring me back to the school!" I called to my mother as I rushed to her side. She was working on a quilt. "Come and hide underneath this blanket," she told me. Naatoyiikakato'si (speaking in Blackfoot) told my mother, "I have come for your daughter to bring her back to the school". "She will go back on Sunday. I want to buy her some clothes before she goes back," my mother told the priest.

The priest was one who always wanted his way and he was not prepared to listen to my mother. "The police will come to get her," he told her and he turned around to leave the hospital. My mother was also very stubborn and she could be mean. Before he was able to exit the hospital my mother had jumped up and hit him from behind!

She hit him on the back of the neck and knocked him down. My mother verbally attacked him at the same time. He ran away, with my mother chasing after him. She brought me back to the school the next Sunday.

I only went as far a grade three. I did not get much of an education. I think I spent more time working at the school than I was learning. It was only when I left and I worked outside that I learned how to speak English.

Another thing which affected our English was that the nuns were French and their ability to speak English was not very good. Consequently, the English we learned was the kind of English they spoke. It was not good English.

I can't really say that the school was bad. In fact it was good. It was only that some things were not right, like the food. It was during the war times when I was in school and we used to take back some of the ration tickets that we got at home. One of these was for sugar.

The students who did not bring back their ration tickets for sugar were seated in the same area and they went without it in school.

I learned a lot of work skills while I was in school. I learned how to cook, how to bake, how to clean house. I worked in the laundry a lot. We had to hang the clothes outside because there were no clothes dryers in those days.

If you behaved yourself you were not punished. But if you didn't you were punished. I think I missed a meal once because I had to kneel down during that meal. I was caught stealing a potato. My mother heard about this and she came and got after the nuns.

I learned how to work. In the process, I learned how to be independent. I had not left the school for a long time when I returned there to work. I worked until it was no longer a residence for the students. Even then I worked for another two years for Red Crow College, where I helped to cook lunches for the students there.

While I was attending residential school we prayed a lot. We prayed in the morning, at noon and in the evening. We were also encouraged to go pray in the chapel in the evening. During Lent we prayed a lot. The nuns and the priests were very devout.

Could my parents have raised me if I had not gone to residential school? My mother was very strict. She and my father were not together any longer. In fact I thought that the man she lived with was my father. It was only later, after my mother died, that I found this not to be the case.

I was headstrong and I often did not listen to my mother and my stepfather. I got into some problems because of this. I don't think that the residential schools can be blamed for the drinking problems which some of our people developed. The priests were always strict and we never saw them drinking.

However, I think that the residential schools can be blamed for some of the loss of our language. They were strict in forbidding us to speak our own language when we were in school. It was there that some of our people started to get used to speaking English. Eventually, we have the situation which exists today. Some have lost their language. Some can still speak it.

One of the priests, Aahsaopi, used to use an illustrated poster to teach catechism. At the bottom of this poster was a depiction of hell. He used to tell us that if anyone joined Iitskinayiiksi they would go to hell. He was against our traditional Indian religion. But he had learned our language and could speak it very well. In fact, he lived to be an old man here and he died here.

The older girls used to pick on the little girls. If a little girl had an older sister at the school, then there was someone to fight for her. If not, then that little girl suffered without help from anyone.

Because of the nature of the residential school and how we were restricted, treats such as candy or berries from home were the source of problems. The older girls would just take any treats which the younger girls got. This happened to me a few times, when some older girls took stuff from me, but I fought back. I was not timid. I also reported these girls whenever they did this to me. I saw some of the students getting strapped. Some were also sent to bed without food. There was some abuse.

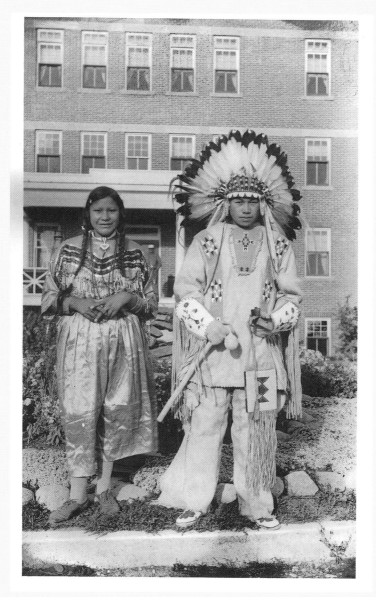

PROVINCIAL ARCHIVES OF ALBERTA/OB.284

Students at St. Mary's School in traditional costume, 1936.

ELDER/SURVIVOR L

1939–1947

I attended the St. Mary's Roman Catholic Indian Residential School from 1939 to 1947. I went to this school because my parents were Catholic. I had to attend residential school because it was the policy of the government of Canada that all reserve students attend residential schools.

The subjects taught when I went to school were spelling, writing, arithmetic, reading and lots of catechism. This was not useful for me later on, not by a long shot.

When I went to school I spoke mostly Blackfoot and very little English. Blackfoot was the only language we spoke at home. At the school we could not use Blackfoot and were forced to speak English.

There was punishment if we were caught speaking Blackfoot. We were not only strapped but we also had to be further punished by doing work that nobody would expect.

There was nothing really which I consider good about my experience at residential school. The regimental style of discipline and the inferiority complex which resulted in us was bad.

I have accepted our traditional spirituality because of its true value in life. However, I still practice my Roman Catholic religion like my parents did.

At residential school I did suffer abuse. I was strapped and slapped in the face many times. A lot of times I cannot remember why this happened. We never could defend ourselves.

I witnessed incidents of abuse done to other students. When I first went to school at the age of seven, I witnessed an incident where a senior girl was horse-whipped in front of the whole student body. This was a very fearful and threatening experience for all of us.

There were other things wrong with residential school. One of these was the food. It was like slop and we were fed this day in and day out. Very few times did we get a decent meal. All the nourishing food was probably eaten by staff. Another was the type of staff who worked at the school. During the eight years that I attended residential school, I noticed that French staff were sent to us who did not speak a word of English. We were expected to learn English from these people— what a joke!

ELDER/SURVIVOR M

1944–1945

I went to St. Paul's Anglican Indian Residential School in 1944–1945. I was around ten years old at the time. Old grandparents raised me and the reason I went to school was because they were told that they would receive a "red letter" (maohksinaaksin) if I was not sent to school. They had no choice but to send me.

When I went to school, I had a name but it was in Blackfoot. I never knew that you were supposed to have a white name and a surname. I was given these two names one day in school. I became very upset at the time.

For two or three years I went to school regularly, then I only attended off and on until I was sixteen years old. My grandfather who raised me died three years after I went to school. My grandmother followed him two years later.

In the lower grades we learned to count, spell and read. It was like kindergarten is today. Because some of the students went to school late, there were all ages represented in a grade. It was the kipitaipokaiksi who were late in going to school.

There were some older students who were more like farmhands than students because all they did was work in the school farm. They were too far behind and too old to be in the classroom. A farm instructor showed them what to do.

I did not learn much while I was in school because I was too busy trying to survive in the environment of the residential school. It seemed that I was constantly dodging staff and students who were constantly after me.

My mind was destroyed. I was told when to get up, what to do and when to go to sleep. Not only that but there were the bullies who were also ordering you to do this and that. I spent all day trying to hide. I got to the point where I could not shed tears anymore. I learned how to cry silently. It was torture from morning to when you went to sleep. Many students hated to wake up.

Blackfoot was the only language I spoke when I went to school. I spoke a very traditional form of Blackfoot because my grandparents were very traditional and they were involved with Niitsitapiaatsimoihkaani. I did not know any English. I went to school with a nice personality. This was during the time when Indians were very kind. They had a lot of love.

The first day I went to school I got into a fight. The problem was I didn't know how to fight. Because I was a kipitaipoka, I was very pampered at home. I was an "only" child and because of this I was unfamiliar with how to play with other children, never mind how to fight! I kept getting into fights because I wouldn't fight back. All I did was try to dodge the other student and I cried. Finally, an older student took pity on me. He told me that the only way the other kids would leave me alone was if I started to fight back. And so I did start to fight back.

We were forbidden to speak Blackfoot. Most of us only knew Blackfoot. So what in effect we were doing was we were keeping quiet. When we were let outside to the playground we felt so much freedom because then we could speak Blackfoot. Many of the other students learned some high Blackfoot words from me because I knew how to speak this way from my grandparents.

In a way, my school experience was good in that I learned how to groom myself properly and I became aware of a style of life which would be useful to me later on. It would have been nice if we had been treated properly but sometimes we were even forced to do what we enjoyed doing anyway. Something I really didn't like doing was "womanly" work like darning socks and waxing floors.

Prayer in any religion is good. Our Indian religion is very powerful. But it is unfortunate that people abuse religion too.

When we graduated from the residential school, we graduated to Indian Affairs. I worked for another grandfather who was wealthy. And I knew other older Indians who were very well off. They had lots of cattle and they farmed successfully. Yet they were not allowed to handle their own money! They were given purchase orders to buy from various government-approved businesses. After a while, they were told that their money had run out. Sometimes I think that they were short-changed. We had to fight with Indian Affairs people all the time because they controlled everything. We were treated like kids even when we left school!

I am an Anglican. I do not want to look down on the churches.

I was very much abused in every way—physically, sexually, emotionally and spiritually. I had no trust or faith in the boarding school. I walked around quietly, silently knowing that I had no one to turn to for help and solace. You had your mother and your father. If you were troubled, you only had to go to your mother and when she put her arms around you, you knew you were protected. I had no one.

One time the principal, Mr. Pitts, asked myself and a friend to accompany him to Glenwood to pick up some potatoes at a Japanese farmer's place. After the three-quarter-ton truck we drove was filled up, we began our trip back. When we reached the old community hall, we saw three boys playing outside whom we recognized as other students. Mr. Pitts asked us who these boys were. We said we didn't know who they were. He knew who they were and he drove over to where they were.

Two of the boys argued with him about coming back to the school and, had it not been for their father, none of them would have returned with us. Eventually, one of them did. Nothing happened immediately after we got back to the school. The next day after dinner our playroom was locked. We could not go outside. We knew something was going to happen.

Mr. Pitts came in and he took off his jacket. He must have been well over six feet tall and he probably weighed around 500 pounds. He yelled at us and said, "Once and for all I'm going to show you who's the boss of this place!" With that he called the student we had picked up at the hall the day before. He grabbed the student by his hair and then he kneed him with one leg. Blood spurted out of the student's face. Again he kneed him with the other leg and more blood gushed out! He really beat him up. We did not want to look. We were helpless.

It was this kind of treatment which created a huge amount of resentment in us. Not only did we have to put up with the staff and the bullies, but we had to also dodge some of the "church goers" who would come down to our playroom after church on Sunday and get after some of the students. It was not a pleasant place to be.

After I left school for good at age sixteen, I helped another grandfather. Then I left the reserve and went to work in the states and in other parts of Alberta. I learned a lot. I realized that I was a capable person. I realized that if only I had had a better childhood I could probably have done so much with my life.

Among the things that I did was I assisted a veterinarian in looking after a herd of 36,000 head of cattle. I learned how to use a stethoscope and I became very adept at detecting what was wrong with an animal. I also worked in a large feedlot. Still later I became one of the first Indian people to begin to work with A.A.D.A.C.

Later, I came back to the reserve.

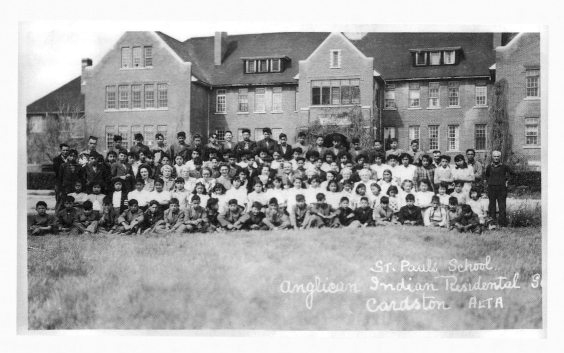

St. Paul's School students, photo post card. Circa 1940s

ELDER/SURVIVOR N

1955– 1964

I was enrolled at the St. Mary's Roman Catholic Indian Residential School in 1955. I was there until 1964. I had to attend this school because the government forced us to go to school. If I had not gone to school, my parents would have been charged. My parents were Catholic. I had to go to this school.

We were taught English, social studies, science, physical education, home economics and religious instruction. I learned discipline and I got an education.

I knew Blackfoot when I went to school. It was the language that we spoke at home. While we were at school, we were not allowed to speak Blackfoot. We were punished if we spoke Blackfoot. I was not punished because I was always scared to do anything wrong.

My school experience was good because I learned how to work. It was bad because I was forced to stay in residential school. It was so lonely without your parents.

I feel good about our people's traditional spirituality and our way of praying. I feel that if you pray in your own language, you understand better. That is better than being forced to get on your knees. However, I still practice my Roman Catholic religion.

I was mentally abused in school in that I was forced to do things I didn't want to do. I got whipped once for not doing what the sisters wanted me to do. Sometimes the girls would get whipped and the teacher or supervisor would make everybody watch. They would sometimes make the girls take off their pants and then they would whip them on their bottom. Sometimes they got whipped on their hands.

I don't like to think back to that time. It is hard to think about the past. It was hard when you couldn't see your parents for a long time. You were forced to eat whatever they gave you, lumpy porridge and green eggs.

ELDER/SURVIVOR O

1950– 1954

I went to the St. Mary's Indian Residential School from 1950 to 1954. My mom and dad wanted me to go to school. Dad wanted me at St. Mary's.

We had religious instruction, reading and writing. This was somewhat useful for me later on, as I could read and write a little.

I knew only Blackfoot when I went to school. It was the language which we spoke at home. However, when we went to school we were not allowed to use it anymore. If we were caught using it we got into trouble. We would have to sit in the corner or do extra work.

What was good about my school experience was that I learned everyday things like cleaning. What was bad was that I did not get a chance to talk with my other family members. I also had to eat what they served us. We also had to wear the clothes that they wanted us to wear.

Our people's traditional spirituality/way of praying is good. It has helped a lot of people. I still practice my Catholic religion.

I suffered bullying in school. The older students would order me around and if I didn't do what they wanted, they would talk mean to me and I would get scared.

An incident of abuse, which I saw, was this one teacher twisting the ears of these small boys and putting them in a corner.

They were very strict at the school. All we did was work and go to church.

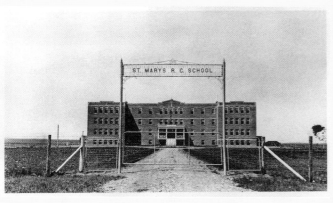

PROVINCIAL ARCHIVES OF ALBERTA/OB.290

St. Mary's Residential School.

TSIINAAKII (MRS. ROSIE RED CROW)

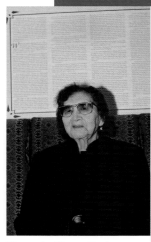

Tsiinaakii (Rosie Red Crow), Kainai elder, who with her late husband, Jim Red Crow Sr., were Ninaimsska and later were also litskinayii members. She joined the holy women's society, the Mao'to'kiiksi, and later the Kanattsoomitaiksi. Tsiinaakii shared some of her wisdom and knowledge about traditional Kainai spirituality, society and history.

ON ELDERS AS COUNSELLORS

We elders are in the high school and we give the students encouragement. I have told you how things were, how the white people's government took advantage of us. You must tell these things also to your children.

In the past, the Bloods were kind people. They helped each other. Even if a person was a bad person, he left his badness behind and helped the younger people, the people just growing up. He would advise and counsel about all different aspects of life. The elder would provide encouragement.

I went very deep into our sacred ceremonials. I was a bundle holder; I was a member of the Horn Society with my husband. I was also a member of the Buffalo Women Society, and I am a member of the Brave Dog Society.

Those who transferred their sacred knowledge to me counselled me: "Whenever you see a fellow member, you will kiss them to show kinship. It does not matter if you see them everyday, you will kiss them. Be patient; do not lose your temper. Even if people run you down and say untrue things about you, be patient. Do not retaliate. Pray for that person who has said these things about you. Try and help each other in whatever you do. Show love to your young people, to the ones just growing up so that they will have the means to survive in the future."

Counselling has been with us for a long time. It was there with those who used the dog as horse and since.

Parents or surrogates of a wayward girl brought her to a person such as this, a counsellor/elder. This elder/elders would talk to the girl, talk to her about the right way. Sometimes they talked to this kind of girl until she cried. These things my father told me.

Child welfare has also been with us for a long time.

Let me refer to my mother, for example, and my uncle. They were still very young when their mother died. Their mother died giving birth to another child. This happened in Montana. My great grandfather brought my mother and uncle home. We're not sure what happened to the baby.

My mother and my uncle were very young when they were brought home. They were raised by this older male relative. They were raised in this way. My mother was fairly old, (about fifteen years old) when she went to school in Dunbow. My uncle missed his older sister so much that he was sent to Dunbow also. My mother said that when he first went to school, her younger brother was with the girls because of his age, and when he got older he went with the boys.

Let's say that that was child welfare. Those who are raised off the reserve by non-Indians miss out. Some suffer because of maltreatment. All these kids should be placed with foster parents on the reserve. We should not send them off.

The holy ceremonial life is good. It makes us kinder people who help others. We help all the people with our prayers. There are some elders who have not followed the sacred way.

Our grandfather Aakaota'siwa (Owns Many Horses) was one of our chiefs.

People would approach him saying, "Aakaota's, I am on foot. Would you lend me a team of horses?" He would say to the person, "There are two over there who look alike. Why don't you break them?" When the person went back later to report that the horses were broken in, Aakaota's would give the horses to that person. This was sharing and helping each other.

My father and uncle used to have a lot of flour made for them. People would come and ask for some flour. My father would tell my mother, "Give them some flour." Maybe the person would say, "I have no food," and my father would tell my mother, "Put some food together for him to take home."

My father told me that whenever someone entered my house, not just to look at that person. "Tell him, 'Sit over there.' Give him some tea. Feed him. If you are just about to begin eating and have not touched your food yet, give him your plate." This is advice my father gave me and advice he got from his father too. This is how my father and my uncle were. They welcomed people with hospitality.

Nowadays, when someone visits, the owner is probably watching television. And he would probably continue watching television.

I had eight children and my cousin Piiaakii had a lot of children too. Everyday we used the washboard to wash clothes. In the winter the washing would freeze when we hung it outside. Then we would have to make a line inside where we hung them again to dry.

We had a lot of sons and we would have to mend a lot of jeans. Then we would also have to sew in padding for hockey clothing they wore. Now they don't do that. We also had to darn a lot of socks. Now when there are holes in a pair of socks, they are thrown away.

When my children were going to school I would clean and shine their shoes after they came home. Today, all the kids wear white runners. But they are not white, they are dirty.

We made our children work. "Help out," we told them. They would take turns doing different jobs. They would ride their horses and herd the livestock. If they had no work to do, they would either go skating or swimming, depending on the season. There was always something that they were doing.

These things are not done anymore. Women do not sew. Now it is the style to have jeans which are torn or worn and which reveal the buttocks or the knees. I tell my grandsons "Aren't you ashamed to show your bodies like that?" They tell me "No. It's the style." What a bad way to dress!

ON BLACKFOOT LANGUAGE AND CULTURE

Let us take Red Crow College for example. They have begun language and culture classes there. The students are strongly encouraged to speak Blackfoot.

I have advocated that in Headstart and daycare, the workers speak to the children in Blackfoot.

Let me use myself as an example. All my daughter-in-laws work. All their children are in daycare beginning at six months. The time they have with their kids after work and before work is not enough. Daycare workers should talk to the kids in Blackfoot.

I work at the Lethbridge Headstart, where the kids learn Blackfoot. When they get home, their parents cannot understand them because they don't speak Blackfoot! I don't want our language to be lost. It needs to survive and continue.

The sacred knowledge is what we cannot discuss. What we see, what is evident, we can talk about; for example, when the Horns dance outside in a circle, or when the Buffalo Women dance inside their lodge. What cannot be shared is the knowledge derived from membership. A person has to be a member to know the information.

The younger people are showing a lot of interest in becoming members in these sacred societies. They are very eager to gain wisdom and knowledge. I have three sons who have joined the Horn Society. My two daughters are members of the Brave Dog Society.

I would like our culture to survive. And I say it will survive, it will last. It is sacred. The Siksika sold all their sacred materials but now they have been returned.

I have a granddaughter who married into the Peigan tribe in Brocket. She went through the O'kaan (Chaste Woman Ceremony) three years ago. This summer she will go through again. These kinds of women are chaste virgins when they get married. They had known no other man before their marriage. They confess to their husbands that they have done nothing to be ashamed of. They are pure. There are other women who perform this ceremony too. When my granddaughter goes through again this summer, she will not eat or drink anything for four days. She will sacrifice herself.

ON EDUCATION, LANGUAGE AND CULTURE

Our language and culture are both very important. Education is very important.

Our heating and lighting we have to pay for. We do not get it for free. We have to have money to get these.

We encourage our young people to get a good education so that they can argue for us. A lot was taken from us in devious ways.

This is our land. The white people came. We did not have a writing system. No one could speak English.

Jerry Potts, whose mother was a Blood Indian woman, was the interpreter. She married a Mexican. They lived in Fort Macleod in a small house. They were storekeepers.

The husband was shot. The younger Potts was taken by the North West Mounted Police and told that they would together look for the murderer of his father. Gradually, he was used as an interpreter by the NWMP. The boy could speak Blackfoot because of his mother but his Blackfoot was not that good because his father had been Mexican. When our people signed the treaty he was one of the interpreters.

Another interpreter was Dave Mills, who was not from here. He married here. He was the father of five children. He was another interpreter.

Another was a man with the last name of Bird. He was from the states and he was an interpreter. At his deathbed he confessed that what he had interpreted had been changed in meaning at the signing of the treaty.

These were the interpreters. We did not write our language. My late father said, "Apparently no one took down notes at the signing Treaty 7. No one. But the pipe was smoked as a sign of trust. Red Crow took some dirt and some grass. He dropped the dirt and held the grass. 'The white man will only live on the grass,' he said. He did not agree to let them dig beneath the grass for them to use. Then our whole land was taken from us."

The first white men here used us for labourers and they used the women for sex. My mother and uncle were half-breeds, half Irish. Your grandmother was also a half-breed. Her dad was Ksisskookitsi. Two of her brothers had a different father but he was from the states and he was white.

Prior to the signing of Treaty 7, the police fired their rifles into the sky and they marched about. They wanted to cause fear in the people so that they would just give up the land. But Red Crow and Crowfoot were intelligent men.

When the police first notified Red Crow that a peace treaty would be signed between them and the white government at Blackfoot Crossing, Red Crow asked that the signing take place in Fort Macleod. When his request was denied, he moved his clan away because he felt badly. Before he left, he left a message which indicated that he would go along with whatever Crowfoot agreed to. However, when he did not immediately arrive at Blackfoot Crossing, the police sent out scouts to find him. Then he went to Blackfoot Crossing. That is how my father told me and his father told him the same thing.

Further, a white man by the name of Akers married a Kainai woman. Then he fenced off an area of the reserve called Aakainaisskoi. This is located near where the Long Time Squirrels live. He fenced off 440 acres. Then he started growing vegetables.

The people said that he was working for his wife, so they did not bother him. He made a living selling his vegetables. Then he would not allow the people near the land. This was where a lot of the herbs and roots used for healing were picked. Also, the wooded area provided the fuel for fire; rocks for sweat lodges were gathered there and there was water. This was a traditional wintering area for the Kainai. Even though this land was never surrendered, it was taken from us in this manner.

In 1970, we got back 222 acres. This was after a long struggle by us old people. The money returned was put into trust. We are working on getting back the other half of this land. We are also helping with the claim for the big lease and the land taken over by the Mormons.

One of our councillors, Dorothy First Rider, is our spokesperson and she has assured the government that we will go after the claim for this land. There are too many Blood Indians today who have nothing.

They are digging beneath the surface of the soil and we do not get any revenue. When this is done on the reserve and some resources are found, we don't get the money. The money is sent to Ottawa.

One time this white man told me: "You Indians are very lazy. You just sit there with your hands held out asking for money… social allowance and old age pension." I told him, "Look here! This is our land. The pension and the social allowance are a small return for the land that you took from us. It is our money and I am not ashamed to take it. It is rightfully ours. Right now we are left with nothing to do. Our land is so small; we have filled up our reserve. We got no jobs on the reserve for all the people. In the past we could trap, cut hay, we had a lot we could do to earn a living. Today, when someone buys cattle to make a living, he has no land to run his herd on. He can't do anything."

It is very hard. There are some of our people who just exist on the reserve. They got nothing. When someone dies and there is a funeral to be held, it is hard for these people to pay the costs. My brother's recent funeral cost $7,000.00. Funerals are very expensive. For our people who own no land, their funeral costs should be covered by the tribe and by social services.

SUMMARY

Not only elders but other knowledgeable people should be available to schools to act as resource people. This is not only for teaching language but also for teaching culture too. The younger resource people need to be persons who have the esteemed traditional qualities such as kindness and generosity. They should be people who know both cultures.

We need to get as much knowledge as we can. We need to instill in the youth that this is vital to our survival. We need to work together and support one another. Cooperatively, we can improve our situation.

We need to give encouragement to our youth and inform them about Blood Indian life. Knowledge needs to be transmitted to our youth. They need to be advised and counselled about all aspects of life.

Our young people need to know about their heritage. They also need modern knowledge so that they can survive in the future. They need to be counselled all the time.

We need to strengthen our kinship ties so that we take care of each other. We cannot allow some of our children to be raised outside where they will have no knowledge about who they are.

It is good that more of our young people are showing interest in the sacred societies. These societies help us to realize our responsibility for others. We become kinder people.

We need to pass on the knowledge of our grandfathers. We must live lives which show that we are real people.

Our young people need to live the natural way. Otherwise we destroy the environment around us. We need to conserve whenever we can. We do not need to consume all the time.

Children need to learn responsibility early.

PROVINCIAL ARCHIVES OF ALBERTA/OB.283

Chief of the Secret Society of the Horn and his wife.

14

GOAL(S)

1. To understand that some students were more severely affected by the abuses of the Indian residential school than others.

OBJECTIVE(S)

1. Students will recognize the abuses which caused some students to lose their self-respect.
2. Students will identify the different types of abuse.
3. Students will learn that parents influenced the outcome of their children's experience at the Indian residential school.

CULTURAL CONCEPT

Indian residential schools on the Blood Reserve affected students differently. Some students were more resilient than others because of the personalities of their parents.

STUDENT ACTIVITIES

1. Students will read/listen to cultural background information.
2. In cooperative groups of four, students will compare the two accounts of student experience at an I.R.S. under the headings:
   - curriculum
   - schedule
   - punishment for speaking Blackfoot
   - learning English
   - perception of what was negative
   - kinds of abuse experienced
   - impact on self-esteem
   - personality of parents/home/background
   - spiritual indoctrination
   - peer abuse.
3. Students will discuss their findings and compare similarities and differences of these to today's situation on the reserve.

EVALUATION ACTIVITIES

1. Students in their cooperative groups will design a poster depicting different types of abuse and how they can be counteracted. These posters will be evaluated for content and message. The best ones will be displayed in the school.
2. Students will interview elders, teachers, parents, health professionals, counsellors and write a two-page paper on why a person with very low self-esteem might easily turn to alcohol and drugs.

RESOURCES

1. Elders
2. Other teachers
3. Parents
4. Health professionals
5. St. Paul's Treatment Centre personnel

CULTURAL BACKGROUND INFORMATION

See Residential School interview —Elder/Survivor P and Elder/Survivor Q.

GOAL(S)

1. To understand that for some students, the I.R.S. provided a steady source of food and warm shelter.
2. Students will understand that there was a price to pay for these benefits.

OBJECTIVE(S)

1. Students will discuss how the problem of bullying was part of the I.R.S. experience.
2. Students will discuss the quality and quantity of food provided at the I.R.S.
3. Students will discuss the importance of good parenting.
4. Students will explain why there were few people who drank in the 1930s and 1940s.

CULTURAL CONCEPT

The traditional diet of Niitsitapi was a high-protein diet. The I.R.S. may have helped to establish a different diet which has had a devastating effect on the health of First Nations people.

STUDENT ACTIVITIES

1. Students will read/listen to cultural background information.
2. Students in cooperative groups of four will speculate on why some families may have needed the I.R.S. to provide food and shelter for their children.
3. Students will compare/contrast aspects of bullying in I.R.S. with bullying in today's schools.
4. Students in cooperative groups of four will research a short paper on the quantity and quality of food served to I.R.S. students. This paper will include how this may have affected the diet of Niitsitapi homes.
5. Students will prepare a poster on good parenting (interview teachers, parents, etc.).

EVALUATION ACTIVITIES

1. Students in cooperative groups of four will develop a quiz on bullying—aspects of it and how it can be stopped. All students will write this quiz later.
2. Students will respond to the question: What price did students have to pay in order to attend an I.R.S. on the Blood Reserve?
3. Students in cooperative groups will develop posters entitled "This Person is a Good Parent Because:____". Posters will include a photo and other appropriate material.

RESOURCES

1. *Kitomahkitapiiminnooniksi— Stories from Our Elders*, Vol. 1–3
2. Elders form list
3. *Shinguiauk's Vision—A History of Native Residential Schools*

CULTURAL BACKGROUND INFORMATION

See Elder/Survivor R and T interviews.

GOAL(S)

To recognize that Indian residential schools affected Niitsitapi society.

OBJECTIVE(S)

1. Students will develop an understanding of alcohol abuse as a coping strategy.
2. The students will understand that the two Indian residential schools on the Blood Reserve created a lot of problems for students.
3. Students will recognize that the Indian residential school institutions on the Blood Reserve did not have high expectations of Blood students.
4. Students will understand that the Indian residential school was part of the federal government's Indian policy of isolation.

CULTURAL CONCEPT

Many former students of Indian residential schools on the Blood Reserve were negatively affected.

STUDENT ACTIVITIES

1. Students will read/listen to cultural background information.
2. In cooperative groups of four, students will discuss the following questions and record their answers:
- What was it about the Indian residential school which caused the shame and suffering, the resentment, the anger, the feeling of helplessness?
- Who do you think betrayed these students? Explain.
- Did the Indian residential school have high expectations of its students?
- What were some factors which helped to make the residential school experience positive for some students?
- The demise of the Indian residential schools was attributable to what new government policy?

EVALUATION ACTIVITIES

1. The cooperative groups will develop questions for a student quiz.
2. Students will take the quiz with an acceptable minimum grade of 90%.
3. Students will review the elders' books and depict on a map the movement of schools and other services from the northern to the southern part of the Blood Reserve.

RESOURCES

1. *Kitomahkitapiiminnooniksi— Stories from Our Elders*, Vol. 1–3
2. *Leap of Faith*, Therese Castonguay
3. *My People the Bloods*, Mike Mountain Horse

CULTURAL BACKGROUND INFORMATION

See introductory pages vii-viii, History of Residential Schools on Kainaissksaahkoyi.

ELDER/SURVIVOR P

1934

I first went to school when I was about five or six years old. This was at St. Paul's Anglican Indian Residential School. I was too young to attend classes. The reason I was there was because my older sister had gone to school and she wanted someone to go with her. Later on my best friend went to school at St. Mary's Roman Catholic Indian Residential School. I wanted to be there with her and so I went to St. Mary's. I went there in 1934.

I did not learn too much while I was in school. When I turned fourteen, I only went to school for half a day. The other half I worked. By the time I left the school, I could only speak a few words of English. It was only years later that I learned more English from my grandchildren.

I learned how to sew, cook and clean at the school. These were useful to me later on when I left the school.

All we spoke at home was Blackfoot. At the school, we were told to speak English. When one of the nuns was around us, we used to make sounds pretending we were speaking English. At least we thought they sounded like English. As soon as the nun was no longer around, we reverted back to Blackfoot. If we were caught speaking our own language, we were physically hit by the supervisor.

What was good about my experience at the school was that I did learn a little English. And I learned how to work, and how to cook and sew. What was bad was that for ten months of the year we were totally under the control of the school. We did not make up our own minds about anything.

We were not served good meals. We were fed the same kind of meals over and over again. Only at Christmas and Easter were we given good food. We also had to steal food because we never had enough. On one of these occasions that I remember, there were seven of us who stole carrots. We were found out and all of our stolen carrots were placed in front of us. One of the students came and bit off a piece of a carrot. When the nun discovered this she hit each one of us.

I believe in our native religion, our native spirituality, in Niitsitapiaatimoihkaani. My father was the keeper of a Ninaimsskaahkoyinnimaan three times. I was raised with our Kainai spirituality because my parents practiced it.

I was baptized in the Anglican Church but I attend all different kinds of churches, including the Catholic, Full Gospel and Anglican. My dad told us never to make fun of any religion because each one prayed to the same God, and that each religion only differed in how they prayed to him.

There were some students who were bad. They would hit us and beat us for no reason. They were bullies. Also, there were two supervisors who were physically abusive. I remember one time one of the nuns really wanted an Indian name so a student gave her the name "Soohkskiina". She was told that it meant, "mouse". Later, when she found out it really meant "big-faced man" she got after us. All of us got a strapping for this.

On another occasion, an older married man had given one of the students a ring. This ring probably belonged to his wife. She came to the school and told Naatoyiikakato'si about it. Eventually he came to our playroom and asked the girl about the ring. She didn't have it anymore because I threw it out the window for her. In spite of her denials to having the ring and to being involved with this man, she got a severe beating. Her beating was so terrible she was knocked out. This was done in front of all of us!

The education I got was very limited. There are still a lot of words I cannot understand. The nuns did not know how to speak English. They spoke mostly in French to each other.

I encourage our young people to learn their language. To them I say, "You're not white, you're Kainai. You should know how to speak your own language."

My own parents never went to school. My father learned how to speak some English when he worked for white farmers off the reserve. In my growing up days there were very few people who drank alcohol. Those who did were frowned upon.

When I left the school, I worked. I did house cleaning. I also worked in vegetable gardens and I stooked grain. We worked a lot. We were not paid that much but we could buy a lot with what we earned in those days.

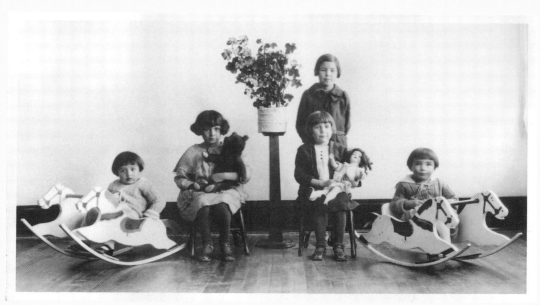

Studio portrait of children from Cardston. (Children from Cardston playing with toys.)

ELDER/SURVIVOR Q

1936–1944

I attended St. Mary's from 1936 to 1944. I was eight years old when I left home. One of the reasons why I was sent to school was because my parents did not want to go to jail. There was a general threat issued by the Indian agent that parents would be imprisoned if they did not send their children to school.

There were only two schools which we could have gone to and one of them was St. Mary's. That is where I was placed.

I spoke only Blackfoot when I went to school. My parents did not know any English and subsequently, neither did we. We were told not to speak Blackfoot in school. If we were caught speaking it, we were punished. We had to kneel in the centre of the playroom where we were most visible. The object was to humiliate us and to make us feel small.

In the morning we had catechism. This was taught by Aahsaopi (Father Levern). Then we had reading and writing and speaking English. In those days we were still fully Indian. When I turned fourteen, I only attended classes in the morning. In the afternoon, I was made to work. Most of the time I was in the laundry helping to wash clothes or I was in the sewing room.

The education I received was not that useful to me when I left school. Our education was not very good. I only went to grade six. Our teachers were nuns who spoke mostly in French. I did not learn that much English from them.

When I left school, I came back home. I began working immediately. I helped my mother at home and I worked at house cleaning and yard cleaning in the local towns. I worked outside the reserve for a while. I worked on farms in Vauxhall and Taber. I also picked apples in the states. Some of what I consider, as a part of a bad school experience, was that we did not learn very much. Some of the nuns were very mean. If we reported to our parents some of the bad things that happened to us, we were later punished for this too. In the end we quit reporting the bad treatment to our parents.

We learned how to sew and how to keep a house clean. These were useful to me later on. When we got older we learned to enjoy the school in spite of the bad things which went on.

Naatoyiikakato'si, the principal, did not hesitate to hit the children. Eventually, he had to be told not to do this anymore. Some of the nuns were kind. Some of them were mean. The mean ones were the ones who made our lives miserable.

We were forbidden to use make-up. As a result I have never gotten used to wearing make-up. We were always served the same food. Many times it was burnt. Always, there was never enough. As a result, we became food thieves because we were always hungry. When we were caught we got the strap.

I was raised with our native spirituality. In fact, at one time I was going to go through the O'kaan. However, because of what Fr. Levern taught us in catechism, I did not go through with it. Generally though, I was not discouraged enough to put away my native spirituality and my native religion.

When my son became a member of the Iitskinayiiksi, I partnered with him. My younger brother had encouraged me to assist my son who needed the help. This is why I have again renewed my involvement in our native religion. I do not run down Christianity. I practice it too. But I also practice our beliefs as well.

There have been some people who exaggerated about what happened to them in residential school. I went as far a grade six. I did not really learn to speak English there.

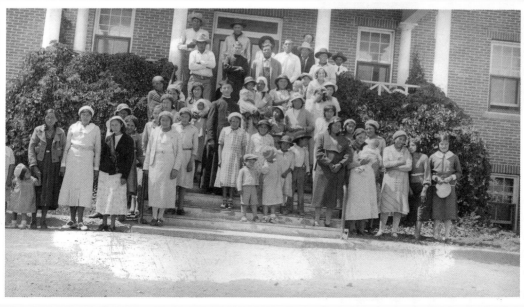

St. Mary's Residential School, 1936.

ELDER/SURVIVOR R

1936

We had to go to school. There was no way that we could escape going to school. I was only six years old when I went to residential school. I did not speak English. I spoke only Blackfoot.

My older sister had already gone to school before I did. Whenever she had to return to school, I cried to go with her. She and I were very close. This is the reason why I went to school so early.

I matured as a result of going to school. While I spoke an English which was very poor, I learned some English. I never experienced being punished whenever I spoke Blackfoot. The nuns who were our supervisors could not speak English because they were French. We could not speak English because Blackfoot was the only language we used at home. We were encouraged to try to speak English so that we and the nuns could mutually help each other learn English.

When I began to understand English and learn to speak it, I still encountered instances when I did not know what a certain word was in that language. By this time, we were being encouraged not to use Blackfoot for certain periods of time. Of course there were children who reported on us. "How do you say this word in English?" I would ask another student. The one who reported us to the teacher would write our names down. But I was not strapped or physically punished. A black star was entered beside my name on a list.

I once went for a whole week without speaking Blackfoot and I was awarded a gold star. My reward, which went with my gold star, was that I went to see a movie in Cardston.

I did not really get a good academic education but we lived in a very clean environment. We were taught good personal hygiene habits. Also, we were instructed on how to maintain a clean home.

It is true that we were made to pray a lot. But that was good. What's wrong with that? Praying has influenced us into living good lives. Today, whenever we gather in a group, we always begin with a prayer.

Today, if I want to sew something, I do not have to go to another person to have it sewn for me. I can do it myself. I have that skill. If I want to have fry bread with a meal, I do not have to ask somebody else to make it for me. I can do that for myself because I know how to cook.

I am thankful to the residential school because I learned some very useful skills there. I learned how to be independent because of these skills.

I went to school in 1936 and I left in 1946. Later I worked there for quite a few years. I learned how not to give up and I have never done that. I have maintained my independence and I always worked. The experience I had at the residential school prepared me for this.

When I first went to school and my parents left me there for the first time, I did not have time to feel homesick. I was too happy to have playmates. My older sister was there already. I did not feel homesick.

My parents would have been able and capable to look after me had I not gone to residential school. But I did need to learn how to speak English. Even though my parents were not rich, they would have been able to raise us at home had we stayed there, in spite of the hard times then.

I was a very playful child. I got into trouble easily. If I was going to be punished for doing something I was not supposed to be doing, I got punished for it. But I did not get punished for nothing, I deserved the punishment.

My shoelaces were never tied. My skirts were always falling down and my hair was never properly braided or combed. This happened because I was too interested in playing and not in grooming myself.

It was the bullies who were the ones getting after us and making our lives miserable. There was one especially who treated me miserably in residential school. She got after me because she thought I picked on her younger sister. She slapped me on the face and she pulled my hair. She was an awful bully. Her presence in the school almost caused me to hate going to school. But then she graduated and the school for me became a whole lot better after she left.

There were not very many people who drank who were my parents' age. I don't recall ever having to run away from my dad or somebody else because they were drunk. The habit of drinking alcohol did not come from the residential school.

Smoking marijuana only arrived yesterday. There were very few who drank. Those who did became well known because there were so few. A girl who became pregnant without being married was also well known because this was not a common occurrence.

The nuns sat us down and they talked to us about our future. "This is for your own good," we were told. They did not tell us to sleep with every Tom, Dick and Harry when we left school! They did not tell us to start drinking alcohol when we left school.

I was still playing with paper dolls when I was fifteen years old. I was not looking at dirty movies. The bad stuff is all new. It only recently arrived. Why blame everything on residential schools?

Look to the future. Prepare for the future. Quit putting the blame on residential schools.

My mother and father talked to us about the proper way of doing things. They were our role models. We were not children who were almost trampled by drunken parents and their drunken friends.

The people still had strong parenting skills in spite of residential schools. I don't agree that parenting skills were lost as a result of residential schools. Those people who have lost their parenting skills lost them because of other factors. One of these was because they were lazy and they did not want to be strict with their children. They did not want to talk to their children.

My parents learned a lot of useful skills when they went to school. My father was able to farm and he was an able worker. My mother knew how to garden and how to can foods. These things they learned when they went to residential school.

Today very few people garden. No one does home canning. People do not have healthy eating habits such as eating vegetables on a daily basis. Too many people eat convenience foods like pizza. They don't know how to eat a healthy diet.

ELDER/SURVIVOR S

1957–1961

I went to the St. Paul's Anglican Indian Residential School from 1957 to 1961. I had to go there. My parents were going to be charged if I didn't go to school. My sister tricked me into going because she said that they showed movies there every night. I thought that would be fun so I went. We were Anglican and there was no other school to go to except the Catholic school.

We were taught math, English, reading, writing and we had religious classes. This was a little useful as I learned some English.

When I went to school I only spoke Blackfoot. We used it all the time at home. Of course, when we went to school we were not allowed to speak it anymore. I got hit for speaking Blackfoot. I was really hit with a wooden pointer. If you couldn't pronounce a word properly, you would get hit. I always dreaded going back to class because I knew what was going to happen.

I can't think of anything good about my school experience. You were controlled all the time. The staff were there just to make you miserable. If it was good I would have continued my education. I was bullied by the other students. I didn't have an older brother so the older boys bullied me. The supervisors punished me for things I didn't do.

I believe in the old ways. That is our way of life. I am very proud of it. I believe and pray in the old way. That's how we were raised from the beginning of time. But I follow the Catholic practice a little and I pray.

I was mentally and physically abused. One supervisor yanked me by the hair because someone threw a spit-ball at him. He pulled me to the bathroom and slapped, kicked and slammed me against the bathroom wall. I had to tell him it was me who threw the spit-ball even though I didn't do it. I had to tell him I did it so that he would stop hurting me. If I didn't, he would probably have killed me. They were very cruel.

I saw kids in the junior dorm get spanked with a scrub brush. If you got up to go to the bathroom and couldn't explain this to the supervisor, he would pull you to the side and hit you with a pointer. This was done to keep the other kids in line. Some kids got bullied all the time and this would happen if you didn't have other relations or family members in school.

Somebody has to be responsible for our suffering. Sexual abuse was there, pain and hurt. If the school had been a good school with good staff, there would be more well-educated people on our reserve. A lot of kids hated school. The conditioning of the residential school caused people to be the way we are now. I hated school.

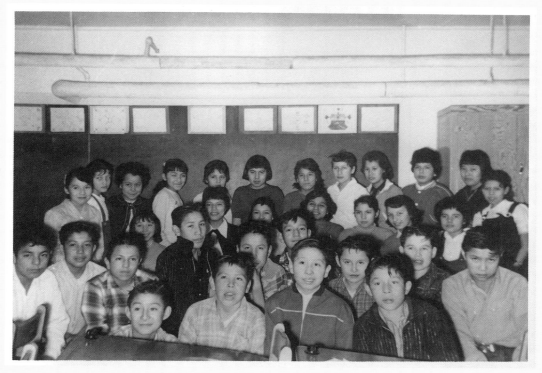

St. Mary's Resdiential School Grade 5 class, 1959.

ELDER/SURVIVOR T

1934–1943

I attended the St. Mary's Indian Residential School from 1935 to 1943. My dad sent me there to get an education. I had to attend this school.

We had English, cleaning, housekeeping, sewing, cooking, reading, arithmetic and spelling. The daily living skills were useful to me later on.

I spoke only Blackfoot when I went to school. I think we were allowed to speak it in school. I don't remember getting hit or slapped but I do remember the first time the sister asked me what my name was and I answered her by giving my name in Blackfoot. She slapped my hand.

My school experience was good in that I learned skills like cooking, sewing and cleaning. What was not good was the bullying of the older girls. They ordered us around and beat us up if we didn't do what they said. They would get after us.

Our people's traditional spirituality way of praying, is a good way if you believe in it. I still practice the Roman Catholic religion.

I was abused by other students when they bullied me. They treated us bad. They wanted us to do things and we couldn't say no. We had to do what they wanted us to do. Because we did, we got into trouble with the sisters.

In this one incident where I saw another student suffer abuse, she was seeing a married man. The man gave her a ring which belonged to his wife. The principal told her to give the ring back and she didn't want to so she threw the ring out the window. The principal whipped her.

We learned a lot. Some people got beaten up. Sometimes the sisters got after us but sometimes I think it was our fault. We got three meals and clean beds to sleep in. They took care of us when we got sick.

TRADITIONAL KAINAI EDUCATION

TSIINAAKII (MRS. ROSIE RED CROW)

ABOUT NAMES

I will tell you first about how my father was given his name, Iitoominaomaahka. In the past we warred with the Cree. In this particular incident, which later became the background for my father's name, a group of Niitsitapi had gone on a raid or a warring expedition.

In this group was a relative of ours who was still very young at the time and was probably on his first raid. This being the case, he was anxious and eager to acquire a trophy of this event. When they finally encountered a group of Cree warriors, he was the first of his companions to reach the enemy and was able to wrest a rifle from one of them.

However, he did not get a chance to enjoy his trophy for very long because an older, more seasoned warrior came up to the young man and took away the rifle. The other members of the war party saw what happened. They all proclaimed that the young warrior "Iitoominaomaahkaw" (he was the one who first took the rifle).

This is how my father was given a war name.

In my own case, I was born at the Sundance. At my birth, an old grandmother by the name of Niinaimsskaakii assisted my mother and helped to deliver me. At around the same time, a female dog of hers had pups at the Sundance.

This grandmother had made friends with some Tsiinay (Atsiina—Gros Ventres) who were also camped at the Sundance. They were in the lodge next to hers. One of the Atsiina women in the group came into her tipi not too long after my birth and requested the pups from my grandmother. "Take my little dogs if you want them," Niinaimsskaakii told her visitor after she heard this request.

The next morning she returned the visit and went to their tipi. Upon entering their lodge, she noticed that the bodies of the little pups had already been killed and were simmering in a pot of slowly boiling water! These people were dog eaters.

When my grandmother returned from her visit, she took me into her arms and talked to me lovingly in the way grandmothers talk to their baby grandchildren. She was praying at the same time and she announced, "So that my little 'daughter' will achieve old age, her name will now be Tsiinaakii."

That is how I was given my name. My name was paid for with puppies!

There was always a basis for the bestowal of a name. There was always a reason for a name. Some were based on war feats. Others were based on dreams.

SIGNFICANCE OF PLACES

Aisinai'pi—Writing-on-Stone

My father told me this about Aisinai'pi. In pre-contact days, when our people lived in the old way, Aisinai'pi played an important part in whether or not a man went off to war. The day before they planned to leave on an expedition, men would go to sleep at the site. They prayed for some kind of sign.

The next morning they would look at the stones. If they were going to be successful, they knew by looking at the stones. The writing also indicated if they were not going to be successful. If it was the latter, they usually turned back. If they went anyway, they were not successful or they were killed.

Ninastako—Chief Mountain

It has only been in recent times that such sacredness has been bestowed on Chief Mountain. In the past it was not like that. True, when people went to the mountains to pick berries or cut trees, they made offerings of tobacco or something else. This was the extent of it.

The same can be said of eagles. In the past eagles were not considered especially holy or especially sacred. For some reason, I don't know what, they have come to be considered more sacred than other birds.

Katoyissiksi—Sweet Grass Hills

My father told me this. He said, "Pinaapitsaikatoyissiwa maatohkoikimmapiiwa (The easternmost Sweet Grass Hill has no pity). Any one who has gone there to seek a spirit helper or sought a vision has been thrown about violently by the spirits there. Aami'tsitsaikatoyissiwa iiksikimmapiipitsiw (The westernmost Sweet Grass Hill has a lot of compassion)."

Recently, at Red Crow College, plans were made for an exchange visit with Browning and other US tribes and to meet at the Katoyissiksi. When we arrived there it was raining. It kept on raining. It was finally decided that we would break camp and leave the area.

The next year similar plans were made, much to my disdain. Before we arrived there it was raining heavily. This time we did not even get there before we decided to turn around. The event was cancelled.

RESIDENTIAL SCHOOL EXPERIENCE

I went to the Roman Catholic School. What is now Red Crow College used to be the Roman Catholic School. I was there for only two years. I had a serious back injury, which only allowed me to be there for two years.

I did not really care for my experience there. Of the time that I was there, I was sent to the kitchen. I would be told to peel potatoes, endlessly. Yet we were always hungry.

Two other girls and myself used to eat some of the potatoes we were peeling. When the nun caught us doing this, we were reprimanded and slapped on the face. This was just because we had eaten some of the raw potatoes.

Where we ate our meals there was a can placed in the centre in which we threw what we could not eat. In the morning we had porridge. There were worms in this porridge. We would throw our porridge into this container. But the nun would bring back the porridge and force us to eat it.

Then we went to the sewing room where we mended clothes. We mended the boys' pants and we used sewing machines to mend socks. This probably caused whoever wore them to get blisters on their feet.

We also worked in the laundry. Even on the coldest days we had to hang the laundry out on the school fences. We did not put gloves or extra clothing on when we did this. On the morning after we collected the clothes from outside, we brought them in and hung them all over the laundry. Wherever there was a spot we could hang something on, we used it.

Our playroom had a cement floor. When we washed it we were given a scrubbing brush and we worked on our hands and knees. We also washed the walls and ceilings. We also had to wash the windows inside and outside. If we hesitated, especially to wash the outside, we were punished.

I saw a lot of children punished for petty things. One of these was for stealing bread. We couldn't help being hungry because of the poor food we were given.

The clothes we were given to wear were very inferior. We bathed once a week. Once a week we changed our underwear. Our dresses we had to wear until the spring. If our parents bought us things like cold cream, make-up and jewellery, these were confiscated and put away.

Our hair was cut above the ears and severe bangs were cut straight across our forehead. We could not curl our hair or wear makeup.

Two of the girls I went to school with ran away one day. They ran to a grandmother's place. Her home was located around Spikskoitapi, close to where Pat Brewer's place is now. The grandmother allowed them to stay one night and she brought them back to school the next day.

Later Piitaotskina, the principal, had the girls brought to our playroom, with only an undergarment on each one. He strapped them in front of all of us. Most of us broke down crying because the strapping was so intense and brutal. They were literally being knocked about.

One of the girls was so severely beaten she had to be carried upstairs to the dormitory. She stayed in bed sick for two weeks, at the end of which she was allowed to go home. Within about a month's time, she died.

I also experienced the strap. The girl who slept in the bed next to mine was scaring us. She was pretending to be a ghost. The nun who supervised us had a corner room in the dormitory. When she came out of her room to investigate what was happening, she thought that I was the one who had been creating the mischief. As I lay in bed, she began to assault me with her strap.

The straps that were used were made from the rubber of old three-ton truck tires. They were thick and heavy. Thick welts formed on my body from the strapping that she gave me. "Why are you strapping me?" I yelled when she was in the act. She paid me no mind but only continued.

Apparently, someone told her next morning that I was not the person responsible for what happened in the dorm and that it had been someone else. That is how I experienced physical abuse in residential school.

The nuns and the priests were mean to the children. We were made to pray every morning and we were discouraged to speak our language. If we were caught speaking Blackfoot we were strapped.

"Do not go to the Sundance. The devil is there. Do not sing your Indian songs, they belong to the devil. Do not go to dances when you go home." We were warned about all these things. I know that this is the truth because I heard them.

If someone stole food in the kitchen, she was strapped for it. We were always hungry because the food we were fed was terrible.

After I suffered the injury to my back, I had to leave the residential school. I was consequently raised mostly by my parents.

If parents did not send their children to school, they were charged and they had to pay a fine. Some went to jail because they did not send their children to school.

I will tell you this story, which my father told me.

A messenger was sent to Crop Eared Wolf who told him that a government official along with a mounted policeman would be paying a visit to the chief on a certain date. The reason for their visit was to establish a law which would enable the government to remove by force, if necessary, any children not attending school.

Crop Eared Wolf indicated his agreement to the meeting. Later he sent a message of his own to a friend who lived in the northern end of the reserve. This friend's name was Manistoko's. In this message he indicated the pending government official's visit along with a member of the North West Mounted Police. "I want you to come to this meeting too," his message said. "You always have something good to say. I want you to speak for me."

On the appointed day, Manistoko's arrived early. He had been there for a while already by the time the government official and the North West Mounted policeman arrived. When they began to talk, Crop Eared Wolf was told: "On this western part of the reserve, you will force the children from their homes for the purpose of attending school."

Manistoko's had just begun to talk when he was interrupted by the government official and told, "You will not talk. Crop Eared Wolf is the one who will do the talking." As soon as he heard this, Crop Eared Wolf replied, "No. I asked him to be here. He will talk for me." The official reluctantly agreed.

"We will make an agreement," Manistoko's said. "My wife has been dead for a while. I have been a bachelor for a long time now. The Queen has lost her husband. She has been single now for a while too. Tell the Queen to marry me. That way we will be the parents of all the people here and all the people across the water. Then you can forcibly remove the children from their homes."

Without any further words, the government man gathered up his books and left. That is how this government person was defeated by Manistoko's. They wouldn't accept Crop Eared Wolf as a suitor for Queen Victoria!

The parents cared for their children. They let them go to the residential schools because there was a law which forced them to do this. The parents knew how to take care of their children. They knew good parenting skills.

Counselling and the concept of child welfare have been with us for a long time. When a child did not listen to his parents, he was brought to people who were noted for their ability to talk to and counsel young people. A child's relatives were responsible for him in case he lost his parents early. To use my mother and uncle as examples, they were orphaned when they were still children. Older relatives raised them.

There is no question about parents not loving their children and not caring for them enough. They placed them in residential schools because they were forced by the government to do so.

I don't think that the loss of parenting skills in today's parents was due to the boarding schools. If you look at my generation for example, we raised all our children. We knew how to raise our children.

The parents today, they didn't go to boarding schools. The reason there are so many problems today is because of a combination of factors. Some of these are: children going to school away from home, lack of prayer, and the use of alcohol and drugs. This is why children hang themselves. Children are taken away from their parents, and this is why there is suicide.

Children, generally, do not listen to their parents today. But they are not all like that. Some young people today are trying very hard to be successful in whatever they are doing.

THE END OF JOSEPH'S CHILDHOOD

GOAL(S)

To understand how alcohol abuse affected Niitsitapi families in the past.

OBJECTIVE(S)

1. Students will discuss the changes in the Niitsitapi home from the late 1950s to the present, e.g. language used, topics, humour.
2. Students will know the difference between the two major societies. Canada and the US in their relationship with indigenous people (laws affecting Indians).
3. Students will discuss the disruption caused by alcohol abuse in the Niitsitapi home.
4. Students will be aware of the physical effects of alcohol.

CULTURAL CONCEPT

Alcohol abuse disrupted the closeness of a Niitsitapi home.

STUDENT ACTIVITIES

1. In cooperative groups of four, students will discuss changes which have occurred on the Blood Reserve from the late 1950s and 1960s to the present. Each group will write their observations on a large sheet and compare these with other groups.
2. Each student will write an account of his/her first experience with alcohol. This experience may not have been personal; it could have been a friend's. How the experience affected the student should be included in this account. Students who feel comfortable doing so, may share their accounts with other students.
3. In cooperative groups of four, students will research the physical effects of alcohol on the body.

EVALUATION ACTIVITIES

1. Have a class discussion on alcohol abuse and its effects on home life.
2. Students will submit a short written paper on why the short story was called, "The End of Joseph's Childhood".
3. Students will submit a short research paper on differences between Canada and the US in their laws regarding Indians.
4. Students will discuss the leading causes of death among Blood Indians and other tribes across Canada.

RESOURCES

1. Kainai elders
2. Kainai Health Centre
3. Kainai Counselling Services

THE END OF JOSEPH'S CHILDHOOD

CULTURAL BACKGROUND INFORMATION

He was fifteen years old. He no longer had to live in the residential school. He now lived at home with his mom and dad, three younger brothers and two younger sisters. He had older siblings but they had their own homes on the reserve. They no longer lived here, but they visited a lot.

Joseph was used to having a lot of family around, not only his parents and brothers and sisters but all kinds of uncles and aunts and cousins. His dad's father was around sometimes too, but his mother's parents were not so frequent visitors. His dad's brother Jack was a favourite uncle. Uncle Jack's house was located about four miles to the east. He was a frequent visitor. Joseph liked listening to his stories. Sometimes it seemed that Uncle Jack and his wife Margaret dropped by almost every morning. They would sit in the big kitchen and visit with Joseph's parents.

When Joseph woke up he always heard his dad and uncle doing most of the talking. Every now and then he could also hear the voices of his mother and Aunt Margaret talking to each other. Many times, the four voices would rise in volume as they laughed about something one of them (usually Uncle Jack) had said. These were usually about funny things which had happened to members of the community. Sometimes they were about different things.

Once he remembered they were talking about two different men on the reserve and how each one had the same English first name. At that time, Blackfoot was still the first language of most of the people and usually many English names were given a Blackfoot pronunciation. For example, the name "Jim". In Blackfoot this name became "Tsiim." How would one distinguish which "Tsiim" was being referred to?

Joseph could not remember whether it was his uncle Jack who had solved it or whether it was someone else. Anyway, one of these men was to be called "Iiksopoisskioh Tsiim" and the other was to be called "Pinaapoh Tsiim." The first name meant "strong-wind-faced Jim" and the second meant "Jim from the east." "Iiksopoisskioh Tsiim" was called that because his face was set in such a way that it looked as if he was always in a strong wind. In the case of the second one, he lived in the eastern part of the reserve.

Many times Joseph went to sleep hearing the voices of his parents talking about people and events. When they talked about people, it always seemed to be about funny things happening to them. Their voices were muffled by his pillows and the approach of sleep. A lot of times he heard them sharing dreams that they had had the night before. He remembered that these dreams were so detailed in their telling.

Throughout most of his growing up years, alcohol was pretty much absent from his home life. He remembered that when he was about five or six years old, there had been a few times when he saw his dad drinking beer or wine, A few times he saw his dad drinking with an older, well-to-do couple who were neighbours of theirs. But he seemed to recall that his dad drank away from their home. However young he was, he remembered that his dad's drinking was a sore point between his mother and father.

Then his dad gave up drinking for a long time. He remembered that this was in the nature of an "aahkoomohsin" or a pledge. These were made so that a sick person would get well or that something would turn out well. They were made between a person and Ihtsipaitapiiyio'pa (The Source of Life). This was not an unusual thing for people to do.

Something which helped his dad abstain from drinking was that Niitsitapi were not allowed to drink alcohol in Canada. If they wanted to drink where it was legal for them to drink, they had to drive across "the line" into Montana on a Sunday, to "tour around St. Mary's" or to "go for firewood" near Babb. Nobody ever just said, "I'm going there to sit in the bar and drink a few beers," or "I want to let loose and drink a few beers." However it happened, anybody who went across usually got drunk.

Joseph and a couple friends of his (who were also his cousins) used to ride horseback into Cardston on Sunday nights. Many times they would see the people coming back from Babb. Almost as many times, they would see the local RCMP vehicles coming back loaded with Indians in the back. Sometimes there was an ambulance carrying dead or injured people from an accident which had occurred on the narrow road between Cardston and "the line."

Sometimes, on Sundays, aawattsiiksi would disturb the peace in Joseph's home. Usually it was an older cousin with friends. At first these were harmless. There was usually just talk involved or, as his mother called it, "aisaohkaani" (foolish) talk. As time went on these visits started to become louder and more unpleasant. Finally, they were outright violent.

Joseph's parents were so patient. They would listen and try to talk as if the other person was normal. They tried to reason and cajole. Later, his dad began to lose his patience and he would argue back. Finally, whenever the older cousin came, his mother would already have prepared a quick escape plan for herself and her two young daughters. She did not want to subject them to the ugliness of these scenes. Usually she drove away and came back much later or the next day. His dad stayed behind to see that there was not too much destruction done to the house.

Joseph usually stayed in his bedroom. In the beginning, the drunks left him alone. He was a quiet person and they seemed to respect that aspect about him. However, after the violence started, he became a target. His cousin would start to vent his anger and frustration on him. Then he became physical and began to throw punches. Thank God drunks usually were not very accurate in their aim. He became an expert dodger, and it was probably only this fact which saved Joseph from becoming bruised and black-eyed.

Later, he dreaded these visits and his life was miserable. On one occasion he was walking home when his cousin accosted him. He was on his thoroughbred stallion and Joseph never knew how he was able to get home without being run over by the mad rider.

Still later, as time went on, Joseph's dad began to be absent from home for longer and longer periods of time. People told his mother that his dad had been seen drunk at different locations. The family did not believe these stories. In fact, they denied them. How could that be when he had gone for so many years without drinking? Remembering all the happy years without having to worry about him, it was unthinkable that it could be so. Then, finally they saw him in all his drunkenness.

After the first time, his dad was no longer shy about being seen drunk. Maatattohtsstoyiisiwaatsiks osimsini. It seemed as if it was all right to be at home drunk.

That day marked the end of Joseph's childhood.

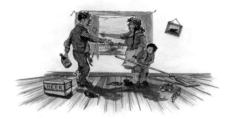

An inter-generational effect of the residential school is alcoholism and physical abuse of family.

GOAL(S)

To learn how alcohol and drugs have generally not been a positive force in Kainai society.

OBJECTIVE(S)

1. Students will read of 5 ways in which alcohol and other drugs have had a negative influence on Niitsitapi.
2. Students will learn how a fetus is negatively affected by a mother's drinking.
3. Students will realize that alcohol was not a traditional drink.
4. Students will learn not to take their lives for granted.

CULTURAL CONCEPT

Every Kainai person has been given a perfect body and a time to live on the earth. Alcohol and drug abuse destroys a Niitsitapi person's body and mind.

STUDENT ACTIVITIES

1. Students will discuss the cultural background information in cooperative groups of four.
2. They will prepare a short group report within a 10 to 15–minute time period. This report will be a reaction to the cultural background information.
3. Each group will present their group report to the class.
4. A community health nurse or health worker will be invited to do a presentation on the effect of alcohol on a healthy fetus inside a pregnant woman's body.
5. Working in their same cooperative groups, students will research one of the following topics:
   • The leading causes of death on the Blood Reserve for the last 5 years.
   • Fetal alcohol syndrome/fetal alcohol effects.
   • Impairment caused to the brain by alcohol/drug abuse.
   • The wonder of giving birth.
   • Teenage pregnancy and alcohol.
   • The effects of alcohol on the body organs.

EVALUATION ACTIVITIES

1. Students will write a short play on a person's first experience with alcohol.
2. Students will write an essay-type exam discussing the negative aspects of alcohol/drug abuse.
3. Students will prepare a poster depicting the lethal aspect of alcohol abuse.
4. Students will prepare a poster on a fetus in different stages of development.

RESOURCES

1. Elders
2. Kainai Counselling Services
3. Kainai Health Centre

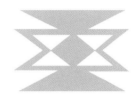

THE UNKINDNESS OF ALCOHOL AND DRUGS ON KAINAI SOCIETY

CULTURAL BACKGROUND INFORMATION

Today, our young people are abusing alcohol. Many live for the weekend when they can run around in their vehicles and consume alcohol. They are poisoning the insides of their bodies. Many have been injured or killed through accidents while under the influence of alcohol. Then there are the bad feelings which are established because of too much boozing and not enough reasoning.

Not only this, but they cause a lot of anguish to their parents and grandparents and any older person who cares about them. We have all been given perfect bodies and a time for each of us to live on this earth. Through alcohol too many of us have spoiled our bodies and our minds. We have wrecked our lives because of alcohol. Too many of our people destroy the quality of their lives.

Other damage which has been caused by alcohol is the damage done to a fetus when a pregnant woman drinks.

A young woman, a girl actually, has not finished school yet. Through alcohol and carelessness she allows the fluid of life to flow into her body. She becomes pregnant. Now she is not one but two people.

She continues to drink and she burns up the brain of the child inside her body with alcohol. She destroys the good life which this little child might have had in the future. When that child is born it is not complete. It does not have all the gifts that is should have to live a proper life. If only there was some way that the mother could have seen her baby before it was born!

Babies are the most precious beings. When a woman has just given birth to a child and she holds it for the first time, there is such a tremendous feeling of wonder and love which she feels for her new relative. A new mother feels like she is standing on top of the world when she holds her baby in her arms for the first time. She is so amazed at the miracle of life.

At that moment in time a woman does not remember the discomfort or the pain of having carried that child in her body for months. She does not remember the pain of giving birth to that child. All she wants now is to love it and care for it and make sure that it grows up safely.

How can a mother burn the brain cells of her child with alcohol when it has not even come into the world yet? How can a mother celebrate the birth of a child when she knows that she has short-changed its life by drinking alcohol while it was still inside of her body?

Anohk aisiikokoyiimmi aniksk pookaiksi maata'konowai'ta'psoka'psiwaiksaw (Children like this become segregated because they will never recover). They will never recover from the effects. This is how damaging alcohol is to the unborn child.

What if this same person had had a normal pregnancy? What if when her baby was born someone came along and poured alcohol into her new child's mouth? She knew that this would have been like administering poison to a helpless child. Would this mother have put up with this? No. She would probably have reacted so strongly against this action. She might have become like a deranged person because she desired so strongly to protect her offspring. So, why did she do it to her child while it was inside her body?

There are some now who pop pills and inject poisons into their bodies. This belongs to another society, not ours. When are we going to use some reasoning? The pills and the use of alcohol have damaged the bodies of so many of our young people. Even some young people now have to watch what they eat because most foods cause acid to form in their bodies. Many too cannot comprehend what we are saying when we talk to them. They just can't think.

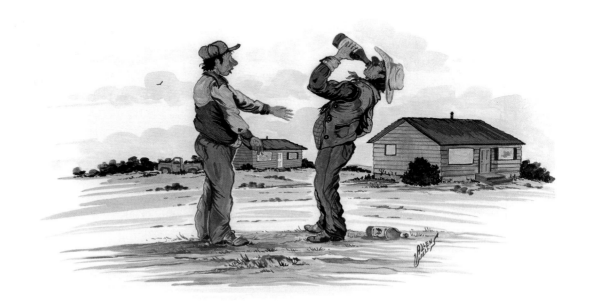

The good life is very different from this. It would be good if they could stop living the way that they are right now. They could live the real life where this kind of pain does not exist. The good life enables us to live a long life, where families and friends are around a long time together.

Some former students and their offspring turned to alcohol to cope with the destructive effects of the residential school era.

ELDER/SURVIVOR U

I share my personal experiences at the St. Cyprian's Residential School on the Peigan Reserve, Brocket, Alberta from 1952–1960. I will attempt to give you a brief history of my background as it pertains to my exposure to residential schools. The majority of my personal experiences in the school were extremely negative, but I do remember having some positive experiences with a particular teacher who was transferred after a brief period of teaching. When I think of her I often wonder why she was transferred. Maybe her kindness was not acceptable. To her I owe some of the peaceful moments I experienced as a child and I will always have a special place in my heart for her.

1952–1960

It is my understanding that my healing will probably take a lifetime. The damage of residential schools is an issue that cannot be reversed so easily.

Before the arrival of the Europeans in North America, Native education consisted of learning traditional skills. This was done by example and observation. The idea that Indian children grew up without education and discipline is wrong. But it can be said that native children grew up without restraint or physical punishment. Instruction and obedience were enforced by moral encouragement. Parents and grandparents taught children survival skills. These skills taught the children how to maintain mental, emotional, physical and spiritual well-being.

Children were believed to be gifts from the Creator. That is why they were given special instruction as well as love by every member of the Indian community.

Both Anglican and Catholic worked hand in hand with the federal government in the attempt to "Christianize" and "assimilate" the native people into the dominant society. Perhaps, the assimilation process would have been successful if they had not segregated natives into residential schools, but instead mainstreamed them into the dominant society. Maybe this flaw was a blessing in disguise.

The children were forced away from their families and put into the residential schools with little or no consultation with leaders or the parents of the children. Laws were passed making education mandatory. The experience was frightening because the children had never been exposed to long periods of separation from their families.

Deep within, the parents had secretly hoped that these institutions would provide opportunities for their children. This is what my grandparents told me. They wanted to believe that these learning institutions would be nice and not oppressive and destructive. But the reality was that these schools were dangerous institutions used to prey on and oppress innocent native children. This oppression became the springboard for later social ills such as alcoholism, poor employment skills and child and sexual abuse.

The separation caused psychological and mental anguish. Children were made to feel ashamed of their culture. The schools failed to establish a quality academic education. Instead, at least two generations of children grew up without the support of a normal family life. They were denied access to a culture, which would have sustained them mentally and spiritually. Compounding this was the virtual inability of parents to do anything to help their children. The federal government had the power to enforce all regulations.

Education was perceived by the native people as being negative because the focus was mainly on the instruction of agricultural methods of farming and ranching. Education to the native people was the development of the whole self, not just a concentration on one aspect of life.

The religious aspect of the teaching created a tremendous amount of fear and confusion among the native children. The new religions claimed to be superior to the Indian religion and accused the Indians of paganism. Native children were systematically brainwashed. They were taught to believe that their culture and values were rooted in evil.

Many of us were routinely punished if we were caught speaking our language, singing Blackfoot songs, or attending any type of spiritual ceremony while we were home. The concepts of "hell" and "damnation" were introduced to us at an early age and thus the seeds of fear and guilt were sown.

Peigan spirituality stemmed from sacred beliefs based on the Creator and Mother Earth as the source of life. The tribes believed in the spirit of brotherly love, in the principle of sharing, in the purification of giving and in the good sense of forgiving. They held ceremonies of thanksgiving and of spring's coming.

The way of life was rooted in a perception of the interconnection among all natural things and all forms of life. They valued the land, the air, the water and the sun. These values were shared not only by members of the Blackfoot confederacy but by all Indian people in North America. All structures and values were developed out of a spiritual relationship with the land.

In the residential schools we were given numbers as a means of identification. We suffered much identity loss and knew little of affection and compassion. We were segregated not only by sex, but also by age groups. Many children were thus denied contact with siblings.

Home became unfamiliar and foreign because we did not know our parents or relatives anymore. Normal stages of puberty and adolescence were stunted because we did not have physical contact with anyone. Our view of life, culture and human sexuality became further distorted by the puritanical influence of the school authorities.

After the residential school experience, it became apparent that many natives were experiencing emotional problems. Many became alcoholics or drifted from the reserves to the urban environment in search of their identity. Many became institutionalized for alcohol-related offences because they fit into the institutional environment. Many were caught between two worlds. Many who had families had difficulties because they had little or no parenting skills.

After I left the residential school, I had very low self-esteem and I was extremely insecure. I had no destination. I had no goals and no sense of identity. In the fall of 1960, my grandparents enrolled me in a provincial school. This was the biggest mistake they ever made. Contrary to what they believed, the residential school had not prepared me for an easy transition. I did not have the proper basic skills to be a student in a public school. I was labelled as being stupid and ignorant by the teachers and students. In no time I was a drop-out.

I began to search for those missing pieces of my life: acceptance, love and affection. I ended up looking in the wrong places and for the wrong things. I ended up in a dysfunctional, abusive relationship with an alcoholic who had also been in residential school. After fourteen years of marriage, I left this relationship because I could not take the abuse and disappointment anymore. I was also an alcoholic by this time.

I knew I had to find something better for my children and myself. I wanted to find out what my real purpose in life was. I wanted to find my true identity. The pain I was experiencing at the time seemed to be an extension of what I had gone through in the residential school, only in a different form.

The reality of the situation was there was no place in this world that was safe anymore. I had been hurting since I was six years old. I wanted so much to gain power over my own destiny. I wanted to be in control of my own feelings, to be a support and caretaker of my four children, and I wanted to gain a focus on my life's pathway. I wanted to leave the residential school experiences behind and I wanted to walk away from all those people who had a part in making my life almost unbearable. I had become suicidal but I somehow never succeeded in ending my life.

Finally, I found a partner who was willing to help me in my search for healing. We have both been sober for almost twenty years. Our children and grandchildren are a blessing. We have found our purpose for life and we have begun the healing process.

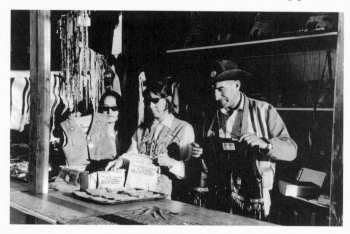

Doris Firstrider, Rachel Weaselfat and Rufus Goodstriker selling crafts. Circa 1970

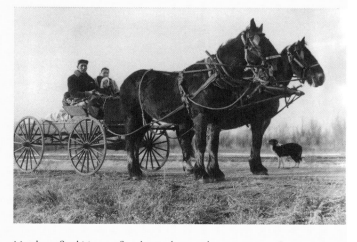

Unidentified Native family in a horse-drawn wagon. Circa 1955

ELDER/SURVIVOR V

1945–1953

I attended St. Paul's Anglican Indian Residential School from 1945 to 1953. My mom and dad were Anglican and they would have gone to jail had I not gone to school. There were no other schools that would take native kids except the other residential school.

We had math, English, science, social studies and spelling. I was thirteen when I went to school. I went to school half a day and worked in the kitchen and laundry for the rest of the day. I also did other odd jobs. The living skills were helpful but the academics was no good. I only learned broken English.

I only knew Blackfoot when I went to school. It was the only language we used at home. When we were at the school we were not allowed to speak Blackfoot. If we did we were punished, strapped.

What was good about my school experience was that I learned some English. What was bad was that the supervisors were mean. They were always yelling at us. They were very strict.

I pray in the native way and I pray in church. I still practice my Anglican faith.

I was physically abused at the residential school. I was forced to eat bad food. I was also strapped or hit. This one girl who was just acting funny to make us laugh was sent to a corner and then the supervisor began to hit her. Another girl who had torn one of her apron strings was forced to wear the apron over her head for three hours.

Residential school was a nightmare. When I think about it I get butterflies. It scares me to think about it.

RESIDENTIAL SCHOOL INTERVIEW

ELDER/SURVIVOR W

I went to the St. Paul's Anglican Indian Residential School from 1958 to 1966 or 1967. My parents were told that if I didn't go to school, I would be sent to a boys' home up north. There was no other place I could have gone. We were taught math, English, religion both in the morning and afternoon. What we were taught was not useful to me because, since I was forced to attend school, I rebelled and I didn't want to learn anything.

I spoke only Blackfoot before I went to school. It was the only language we used at home. However, when I got to the residential school, I could not use it anymore. If we were caught using it, we would get whipped or sent to the dorm.

I can't find anything good about my school experience. It felt like being in jail. The way that the teachers and the principal treated us was very bad. They were mean and cruel. If we were caught talking Blackfoot, we were locked up in the dorm.

I feel alright about our people's traditional spirituality. At school we couldn't practice our traditional ways or we would suffer. I do not practice the Anglican religion.

I was physically abused in school. I was strapped. One time a bunch of kids were running up the stairs and I was the last one. A supervisor tripped me and I hit one of the pillars. I have a scar above my eyebrow because of it. I saw a supervisor beat up two students because they couldn't say, "holy night, silent night". They kept singing it in Blackfoot.

We were treated pretty bad. If we had been taught slowly in the white man's way of living and learning, there would be more well-educated reserve people today. There was lots of sexual abuse, which caused hurt and pain to many students. Native people rebelled and the government should be held responsible for all the suffering of the reserve people.

1958–1967

ELDER/SURVIVOR X

1960–1961

1965–1967

I attended both residential schools on the Blood Reserve. I was at St. Paul's for a year beginning in 1967. I was at St. Mary's in 1960–1961 and again in 1965–1966. My mother was ill and she sent me to these schools. I could have gone to Cardston, which was the nearest town.

We were taught religion, math, English and social. They were not useful to me later on after I left school.

I spoke mostly Blackfoot when I went to school. I knew very little English. We spoke Blackfoot at home. At the schools we were not allowed to speak Blackfoot. If we were caught speaking it we were punished. We had to kneel down in a corner and pray for forgiveness for one or two hours. We could not move.

What was good about my school experience was that I met other people. What was bad about the schools was that they were unreasonably strict.

I think it's important to believe and be respectful about our traditional spirituality. I still practice the Catholic religion.

I suffered physical and mental abuse at the residential schools. Because I am left-handed, the teacher told me I would go to hell. I was forced to use my right hand and I was slapped. I had my hair and ears pulled if I didn't. I was real scared.

Other students were also abused. My stepsister was acting silly and she got into trouble for being mischievous. She was hit on the hands, wrist and arms. One girl was stripped and put into thin pajamas and made to lay on a mattress in the middle of the room. She was then strapped in front of the other girls. Often we were sent to bed hungry. Sometimes I let my sister sleep with me because she was so scared. She would wet the bed and I would take the punishment because I didn't want her to be punished.

If we had been treated better and given a better education, maybe I would have learned something. Three years of my life are a blank. I don't remember anything. Sometimes I think maybe that something bad happened to me. I know it did to others.

ELDER/SURVIVOR Y

I went to the St. Mary's Indian Residential School. I went there from 1960–1961 and again from 1965–1966. Our family lived close to the school so I went to this school the first year. The second time I went to school there was because my mother was in the hospital for a long time and my dad couldn't take care of us. There was no other place I really could have gone to.

1960s

We were taught math, social and English. I really didn't learn anything so the teaching was not useful to me.

Blackfoot was the language we used at home and, therefore, when I went to school, that was the language I spoke. We were not allowed to speak Blackfoot in school. If we did, the supervisors would get mad at us.

There was nothing really good about my school experience. I had to eat what was served to us. Even if I was throwing up in my bowl, I had to eat the food with my vomit.

I wasn't raised with our traditional spirituality but I don't mind it. You get a good feeling when you pray. I don't go to church anymore. I do my own praying.

I was physically and mentally abused when I was in school. There was also sexual abuse because some of the teachers touched us or rubbed us where they shouldn't have been.

One time in class the teacher asked me to do a math question on the blackboard. Another student and I got up to do the problem. We both got the right answer. The teacher beat up the other student cause he said he got the wrong answer. He grabbed me by the hair and pulled me to the blackboard even though I got the right answer. Whether you were right or wrong, you got hurt.

One of the classroom teachers would grab this girl by the hair and bang her head against the desk. I didn't actually see her do this but I could hear her head banging against the desk. I didn't see her cause I was too scared to turn around and look. The other kids say they saw him doing this.

At another time, one girl had to use the bathroom. She kept raising her hand to get permission to go but the teacher ignored her. When the teacher wanted someone to get up and read, she picked that girl. The girl had waited so long that when she stood up, she peed in her pants. I felt bad for her.

I wish that bad things had not happened to the natives when they went to school there. It destroyed a lot of lives and families.

111

ELDER/SURVIVOR Z

1958– 1969

I attended the St. Mary's Roman Catholic Indian Residential School from 1958 to 1969. My parents sent me there. I felt I had no choice. I didn't know I had other options.

At the time, all the subject areas were offered in the curriculum. Even though this was the case, what I learned was not really useful when I left the school. We had to do a lot of the work on our own. A lot of the time I was lost; there was no individual help for students. I didn't know how to ask for help.

We spoke Blackfoot at home. When I went to school we were not strictly forbidden to speak Blackfoot.

What I learned at the school which was useful to me later on was discipline. I also learned how to clean really well. On the other hand, the school was the worst place to gain any kind of self-esteem. My self-esteem was nonexistent and I was painfully shy. I think this still lingers to today. I was quiet, I didn't like to bring attention to myself. I blended into the woodwork. After I left the reserve I realized that I could have done a lot better when I was in school.

When I worked at Pound Maker's Lodge was when I gained a lot of personal growth and self-esteem. Over the years I have attended different workshops which have also helped me. An example is "Vogue Models" through Casablanca.

I have tremendous respect for our people's traditional spirituality and our way of prayer.

When I attend a church function today, I go out of respect, such as when a nephew or niece is baptized. Otherwise, I am not a practicing Roman Catholic. More than likely also, I would probably request to be buried in the same manner as my parents were when I die.

I wasn't sexually or physically abused when I went to school. The abuse I got was from the other students. I was very fearful of getting called on in class because I didn't want to be wrong. I did not want to be the object of ridicule from the other students.

I witnessed an abusive incident after some girls had run away from the school. When they were caught and brought back they were strapped. This was very traumatic. I felt for the girls and I was quite shaken by the incident. All of us had to gather in the dorm. After the girls had put on their pajamas they were strapped. The strapping was administered by the principal who was also a priest.

The first impression I got when I went to school was this great big room with so many girls in it. It was very intimidating. I think I was five years old. I was going to be six that November. Then, I didn't realize that my family was materially poor. But the other girls told me we were poor. But I never felt poor.

My home life before I went to school was in isolation. We lived isolated from others. We didn't see a whole bunch of people.

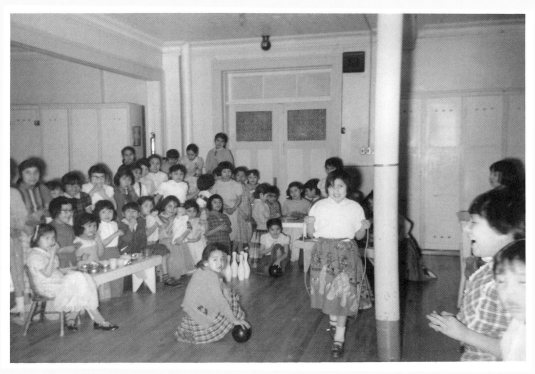

St. Mary's Residential School, 1959.

RUFUS GOODSTRIKER

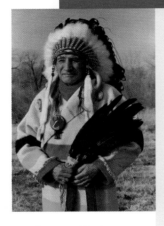

Piinakoyimm (Rufus Goodstriker) is a respected Kainai elder and healer. He is a past member of Iitskinayiiksi. He was an outstanding athlete in rodeo and boxing. He was head chief of the Kainai from 1965-1967. He is a descendent of a famous Kainai leader by the name of Piinakoyimm.

My name is Piinakoyimm. When did the people start using naapiaohki?

Our grandfather, our late grandfather Spitawa, Iinakspitawa, Chester Davis, was the husband of Issksipoohsapawaawahkaawa. From Fort Benton in Montana all the way to Rocky Mountain House he was a supplier for food and alcohol. Beginning in the 1860s, alcohol was introduced to our people here. That is why there is a location called Iitoka'poyi'nitspi.

The white people who lived at the forts, whose homes were built inside the walls of the fort, were the whiskey traders. The people traded horse hides, buffalo hides, horses and whatever else they could trade for alcohol and rifles. It is said that when the pile of hides equalled the length of a rifle was when they had enough to trade for that rifle. It was called an "even" trade.

The people enjoyed trading. They wanted the rifle because it made hunting easier. But they also traded a lot for alcohol. Many of the people were killed during this time. That is why Fort Whoop Up is called Iitoka'poyi'nitspi.

This fort figures prominently into another story regarding Onistaahsiisoka'simi. Apparently this person was an early panhandler of Forts Whoop Up and Kipp. "My children, I am thirsty. Give me a drink," he would tell the traders.

They put up with his behaviour for a while. However, they got tired of him. A special bouncer was hired to fend him off especially. This person was a big black man noted for his strength. "You will have to wrestle this person first," the traders informed him. "Give me at least one drink first," he continued to beg. They gave it to him.

"I will give you four chances first to unseat me and then it will be my turn," he told the black man. The other person agreed and he attacked Onistaahsiisoka'simi. At each attempt, Onistaahsiisoka'simi grunted and somehow prevented his body from being lifted. Then it was his turn. "Okay son, it is now my turn," he told his opponent. In no time he lifted the other man and threw him down on the ground. The force of the fall was so great, one of his legs was broken when he hit the ground.

Onistaahsiisoka'simi had some kind of powerful medicine! He loved to drink and he was known as a bad drunk. When others knew he was into the bottle, they left him alone to avoid his mean temperament. His relations with the traders went from bad to worse after one of his drinking episodes.

Apparently, the alcohol, which the traders were trading with, was being mixed with tobacco and other substances to make the "whiskey" more potent. It was a poisonous concoction.

The traders at Fort Kipp formulated a plan to kill him. An ignorant Onistaahsiisoka'simi went to this fort and asked for his free drink. The traders got him drunk and beat him up. Thinking they had succeeded in killing him, they threw him into a root cellar. A short while later they heard him singing outside. He was not dead! Some power, he must have had.

They "killed" him again with the same result as the first time. By the third attempt they were really frustrated. "We kill him but he seems to come back to life. Let's put him in the river and drown him," they said. The weather became their accomplice in this next attempt because it was now winter and the river was frozen over.

They tied a rope around his neck and brought him to the frozen river. At certain places here and there the river did not freeze. They dragged his body to one of these holes in the ice and pushed it into the frigid water. To make certain that the body really went under the ice, they used a long branch to push it in.

A few months later the weather had changed and the spring run-off was already over. A Siksikaikoan travelling on the Sun Road between Kainai and Siksika happened upon the body of Onistaahsiisoka'simi. It was lying in the debris of a sandbar.

"Tsaa, there's a body lying here!" he called to his companions. "It is the one called Onistaahsiisoka'simi. They say he liked to drink so let's give him a drink," he said. They held the corpse's mouth open and poured some alcohol in. This offering of a drink was more or less a gesture of respect to the fact that the dead person had enjoyed his alcohol. After the second time that they did this, they felt the body move! They fled in all directions. Had they given him more, would he have become a pa'ksikoyi?

The reason I have told you this story is to tell you about the bad effect alcohol had on our people beginning in the 1860s. That is why the name litoka'poyi'nitspi was coined to name that area. Many of our people died there as a result of alcohol.

Not only did this happen but our people were swindled by these traders while they were under the influence of alcohol. It was only when the Red Coats (North West Mounted Police) arrived that there was a force to stop the harm that these traders were doing here. The traffic in bad alcohol was stopped.

Apparently, some of our members yearned for the feeling of being intoxicated. There were stories of people afterward who drank huge amounts of tea to get to this state. After they had been drinking this tea for some time, they began to sing their songs.

Later on the people who drank in our tribe were known. "Watch out for that drunk," people warned each other when they saw such a person anywhere. There were not that many people who used alcohol later, and so the ones who did stood out and were noticed.

By this time, the priests and police had arrived and were settled. Most of the children of the tribe were all in school. People who were intoxicated at dances were noted "Ayaawa iitattsiw"(so and so was drunk there).

At these dances, the children kept close to their parents. In fact, the mothers set their bedding around them and, as it got later, the children slept on these. They did not run around and bother anybody. They were warned that the aitapiooyi (people eater) would get after them if they did not behave properly.

In fact there was a special dance for this person, aitapiooyi. He wore a special costume to hide his real identity. The children were afraid of him. Other characters whom parents used to scare their children into proper behaviour were aawaahkanisstookiaaki (the ear piercer), or aotsiipihtaki (the dunker) or aisstsipisaaki (the whipper).

In 1920, there was almost a huge conflict among our people when the "Soldier's Settlement" referendum was conducted. This involved the sale of a large part of our reserve land. The "yes" (to sell) side was in the majority, according to the government documents.

Some of our leaders who lived on the western part of our reserve got together and collected a fund. With the money they collected, they hired a lawyer and asked that a recount be done of the votes in the referendum. Many of the votes were not valid, as there were under-aged people who had been allowed to vote. Other discrepancies were found. Thus the sale of the 40,000-plus acres which would have been sold in the "Soldier's Settlement" was not allowed.

Where the Blood Tribe Agricultural Project is located is about where the "Soldiers Settlement" land would have been located. In fact, if we are not careful and make sure that B.T.A.P. is successful, we might still lose this land today.

I have not heard of a medicine which will make a person stop drinking alcohol. When a person drinks alcohol he thinks, "I will drink from this." When he has made a home for this alcohol in his body, it is up to him to decide "I am going to quit." There is no medicine for it.

I am a herbalist now. It is mysterious how some things work.

I went to Lac St. Anne where a long-time friend of mine lives. I was treating him for some health problems he acquired because he drank too much. His kidney and his spleen were rotting from alcohol abuse. He asked me for some of the medicine I give him each year.

I get my medicine in the mountains and it is the food of the grizzly bear. I call it licorice root. I gave him all that I had.

Our medicines are sacred. The Creator placed them here. All the land animals and birds use these medicines too. When someone is given the knowledge to use a medicine, the power must be respected. It is sacred.

If you are given this knowledge, use it with wisdom and with care.

I do not smoke but I always have tobacco with me. Whenever I come upon a plant which I want to use, I make an offering before I take it. "Oki Ksaahkommiitapi. Aamostsi nitaako'tsihpi. Nitaahkamohtsissitapiiyaw. Iitstsi'p aisttsiistomii. Nitakohtotoi'tsikataw" (Oki Earth People. I am going to take these. I might have need for them. Someone is sick.).

In 1968 this old lady adopted me as her son. Her name was Iipisowaahsiiyiitaopi. She was the one who instructed me on what to do. "Offer something before you take from the earth," she told me. When to pick them and how to dry them, she included in these instructions. What I was to use them for she also showed me. "Do not try to make personal gain from this," she warned me.

Sikssipistto was another person who adopted me. He was from North Dakota. He also told me, "Respect your power to heal. Do not try to make personal gain from it. After you have succeeded in curing some people of different illnesses, you may become tempted to charge people. This is why I discourage you now from making personal gain from it. Even if a penniless person asks you for help, you should go ahead and help him without expecting to be paid hundreds of dollars for this.

If you begin to ask for a lot of money in return for your healing, the holy ones will come and they will take the healing part of your power away. They will do this because you will not have lived up to your contract to heal people. It was not given to you to make you a rich person. Whatever people can afford to pay you is what you accept. You should not expect to become rich from your gift to heal."

There are many former healers now who are unable to heal. They are using their powers in other ways. You can find them at powwows, for example. "Here is a hundred dollars for you to destroy that singer's voice right now," someone tells one of these. This is done because there may be a prize of $2,500.00 for the champion drumming group.

There is a lot of this happening, where former healers can only do wrong now. Their power to heal was taken back and all that is left is the power to do wrong. They can only hurt people. Many Indian people suffer from isttsikaanitapiisini; they do not like to see others succeed.

This goes back to the way we are raised and the values that we have. Loving, caring, sharing and understanding are four values which a husband and his wife are supposed to instill in their children. We tend to overdo the caring part. Unlike people on the outside who only are concerned for themselves, we care too much to find out what everybody is doing. Any little thing that happens in our communities is known by everybody within a very short time.

If someone kills a deer, the meat from this deer will not last beyond two days. This is because the meat is shared with everybody. The same with the herbs for healing. They have to be shared.

The birds migrate each year. They leave and they come back. Sometimes while they are in transit, they may become ill. They will land on the ground and search for the roots and herbs they need to cure their ailments. They cure themselves. The same applies to land animals. It is holy. It is sacred. That is why we have to respect it.

With regard to alcohol and my friend from Lac Ste. Anne who had asked for the herbs I used to treat his condition, I agreed to his request. I gave him all of my medicine.

Shortly after this I was invited to participate in a sweat. A group of other healers had invited me. We were all seated waiting for one more person. While we were seated I smelled the aroma of licorice root, of the kind of medicine I had given away! I went into the woods and within a very short time, I found it. I dug up all six plants.

By this time the person we had been waiting for arrived and we went into the sweat. The sun was still quite high in the sky; it must have been about three o'clock. When the sweat lodge had been opened a second time, I heard an old Cree man speaking, then a Cree woman. We went back into the lodge.

The host of the sweat who sat foremost inside the lodge told me about what had been stated in the conversation. He said, "You heard those two people talking. One of them was my brother. They know you. They know that you are a compassionate person. They know that you have become this way because of your gift to heal.

"They have given you two more medicines to use in addition to the medicines you have dug up and which are outside." By this time the aroma of my medicine had spread and the air around us was permeated with it. One of the new herbs was to help a person stop smoking.

I was to cut up the medicine into a whole number of smaller pieces. When I was in a circumstance where I was tempted to smoke, I was to chew on a piece of it. It would help to curb the urge to smoke.

The person who wants to quit drinking may find himself in a tempting situation when he passes a bar and he smells the perfume of alcohol. "Oh, one won't hurt me," he says to himself, especially when his friends appear and urge him to come into the bar for a drink.

It is the responsibility of the person who has indicated his desire to quit drinking. When he sits down with his friends who are going to drink, he needs to put a piece of the medicine in his mouth. "Oki, my friends. I have drunk with you a long time. I now have three children of my own. I want to quit drinking. Alcohol has not done me any good. I have suffered from the use of it. I thank you for inviting me." This is a good way to say "No."

Many of our so-called friends we meet only when we're going to drink. They are our friends then. Where are they when you are lying in the hospital suffering and dying of cirrhosis? It is your parents and your family who are going to be looking after you then. Not your so-called "friends."

Alcohol has done a lot of bad things to us. False friends have been created because of it. At weddings where there is always a party afterwards, vehicles get dented every which way and many guests end up fighting with each other. These are all friends. They must be friends. Alcohol is dangerous. That's the way it is. It was not given to us. It came by way of the white people.

TRADITIONAL PHILOSOPHY

In the past, all the people were very close to the one we call Creator, the Source of Life. He placed all the medicines here on Mother Earth. The birds and the land animals still know these medicines. We do not know them anymore. Instead we have been converted to the white man's medicine.

We are in a precarious time now. Our treaties are being undermined and the medicine which is covered under these treaties will no longer be free to us. At that time we will realize how wrong we were to neglect the knowledge about our own medicines.

These medicines which I have on display here, they are not very many. I use twenty. There are fifty-nine medicines here. The Creator gave them to us. Those old men and old women who went before us knew how to use every one of them.

For example, in a camp where someone was sickly from a stomach ailment, he was told to seek a particular old woman who was noted for curing these. Or, if a person had a headache, he was told whom to seek for help. Various individuals were given the power to heal. There was no such thing as "office hours" for treating illnesses! All they realized was that they were healers and that someone needed their help.

It is such a pity that we no longer possess the knowledge of our ancestors. They had a treatment for all kinds of illnesses. They harvested their herbs and roots at the right times. They used these when the need arose. They didn't rush to a clinic where they got many different kinds of pills to swallow. All the different kinds of medicines are there; they are just waiting to be picked for use. But all we do is rush to a clinic, rush to a clinic.

It is evident that the natural medicines work.

All the land animals and the birds treat themselves with these natural medicines. They know how to use them. How we acquire the knowledge to use these natural medicines is a sacred process. Those people who were noted herbalists and healers went through a lot to acquire their knowledge. In most cases, they went through some suffering to acquire the medicines.

Herbalists/healers develop their gift to heal through searching. I am that way myself. One method which helps me in this is meditation.

Naatoyiitapiiksi help us figure out how we will use these medicines.

SPIRITUALITY

What goes on at the Sundance is very holy. Opposite of this is what happens at the Indian Days grounds. There, there is drinking and the people dance for money. It was not our culture to be paid to dance our dances.

At the Sundance, Iitskinayiiksi and Mao'to'kiiksi camp there for two weeks out of the year. Members of these two societies pray and paint faces during these two weeks. Tribal members who have pledged to participate in an event at the Sundance complete their pledges.

They work as healers during this time. Their work is similar to aisimisstsiw. Aisimisstsiw is what I am. A person who has an ailment will come to me and explain what is bothering him. Then he requests that I provide a cure for this ailment.

Should we lose our treaty rights, which includes free medication, those who really have a dependency on these will suffer greatly. These medicines are very costly, they are not cheap. Many will not be able to afford them. There are very few who can claim that pills have cured them of an illness. The effect of our medicines we can see. They help a person to become well.

The three major areas which need looking after are water, oxygen and the blood. There are four parts of the body which also need to be treated. These are the head, the chest, the stomach and the pelvis. In comparison to western medicine, for example, there is an ear and nose specialist, an abdominal specialist and a throat specialist. Each doctor takes apart a sick person according to his or her specialty. They make a lot of money from one person's body. They don't doctor holistically.

Native healers, on the other hand, will paint a person's face, and they will pray while they are in the process of healing, They do not divide up a person's body but rather treat the body, mind and spirit of the person.

Look at my braids. There are three strands. Look at braided sweetgrass. There are three strands in a braid of sweetgrass. Why is this?

When we are being given the power to use a medicine for healing, we are told to value the knowledge that we are getting: "This is when you will gather them in the year. This is how you will prepare them before you use them. This is what you will use them for."

In the short past, at the Castle River Wilderness Camp for prison inmates, I asked for help to gather some of my medicines. I asked this group made up of members of different tribes to gather some wild rhubarb and bear root for me. In return, I promised I would contribute to a general fund which helped to pay for some of their personal needs.

Most of these inmates were in jail for alcohol-related offences. Many enjoyed alcohol. In the interval before I picked them up and after they had gathered the rhubarb, they became curious. They boiled a bunch of the rhubarb and many of the inmates drank from the brew. Before morning of the next day, all of these men were sick and they were all in the hospital!

I use seven different types of sage. Depending on what kind of sage it is, I will use it for smudging or for incense. Sage is used mainly to purify.

If I went to a Mao'to'ki or Iitskinayi and asked to be purified, they would use sage and ochre for this purification. Or, if someone had just had an all-night smoke and he wanted to leave an offering, this offering would include sage. This is to purify that offering, which is why it is placed with it. Sage is very important, it is a necessity.

This medicine that I carry, it has sage in it.

Anyone who wants to collect sweetgrass should be mindful about thanking the Creator and praying before they pick it. When they bring it home, they braid it. Most people who pick sweetgrass use it properly. But there are those who want to use it to get alcohol.

"Let's go and pick sweetgrass and sage. We can sell it to get some money for booze," they say. That's not right. That's not respecting the use of that plant.

I will pay for sweetgrass but I don't sell it. I use it all the time.

We offer prayers when we are going to remove a medicine from the earth. We pray again when we prepare the medicine. We instruct whoever is going to use it to pray before they use it. When you are finished using a medicine, you take it outside and pray again to the Creator, to Mother Earth and the other earth spirits thanking them for the use of it. You do not throw it in the garbage, nor do you burn it. You recycle it back into the earth.

I give all of these instructions to anyone who comes to me for medicine. Many people come to my home for remedies. I do not have a sign on the road saying "Doctor Goodstriker helps people with stomach problems." Many people come to me for help. Some non-Native people often ask me if I can give them my card. No, I don't have a card. I am not running a business!

People seeking help often ask me how much I charge. Whatever a person wants to give in return for my help is what I accept.

ADVICE FOR YOUNG KAINAI PEOPLE

There is a growing problem with prescription drugs in southern Alberta. I was at a meeting in northern Alberta not too long ago and this health worker made the point that the worst case of prescription drug abuse was in Lethbridge, Alberta. This means Bloods, Brocket and Lethbridge.

It's not funny. Taking all kinds of hard drugs into your body is not right. They are dangerous. With alcohol, we can see immediately how bad it is for you when we witness a person's hangover. With some drugs, the result is not so evident. Some forget to wake up.

Alcohol is not for us, it is bad. I used it myself; I know what it's like. The advertising being done by breweries at sporting events seems to indicate that after your hockey game, for example, have a big drunk! When I coached hockey in the past, one of the conditions I had for my players was that there was no partying.

The same applied when I coached boxing. There was to be no drinking. I trained a number of Golden Boy champions: Norbert Fox, Edward Soup, Eddie First Rider and Charlie Small Face

In 1962, when we won the aggregate trophy of Alberta, I was really proud. In the last night of boxing in Edmonton, there were supposed to be twelve bouts in the final night. What made me so proud was that half of the card were Blood Indians versus the whole Western Command.

There was only one outsider—Westside Edmonton had one boy. The rest was Princess Patricia Army, Wainright Army, Currie Barracks Army and the whole Western Command. We won that aggregate trophy. Morris Holy White Man was the last one to fight Colonel Macleod and he beat his opponent. I was so proud! My goal had been to coach young boys until we had won the aggregate trophy. When we won that year, I had reached my goal.

Later on I coached some boxers professionally, but they began drinking and it was not worth it. They could get hurt and I could have gotten the blame. It would have been really bad if I drank with them.

Look at all our wonderful athletes. Look at Jim Thorpe, a world-known athlete, he died of alcohol. Tom Long Boat also died of a sickness related to alcohol. These were outstanding Indian athletes.

Why is it we get that way? Why are we so visible when we are drunk? At the Calgary Stampede, we may be sitting in the bleachers. Another Indian passes us by staggering drunk. All the whites see him and think "See, that Indian's drunk!" Another drunk comes along but he's white and it's "Boy, he's having a good time!"

Freddie Gladstone, Jimmy Gladstone and Pat Wolf are all doing a big show for the Indians in the rodeo. But this one Indian who is drunk wipes out all the "bigness" that these other ones have done.

I saw changes occur in the 1950s. In 1962 the government came in and told us that religion was not to be taught any longer in the classroom. That is what is missing today, prayer in the classroom. We are doing our own praying in our schools and the government can't do anything about it.

In 1950, when I worked as a constable on the reserve, I organized square dancing for the young people in the various communities. The young people had a lot of fun. Their parents accompanied the young girls to these dances.

Prior to the 1960s, the people broke their own land, they grew their own crops and gardens, raised cattle and chickens. No one was rich but the people were independent. They looked after themselves.

Then the government brought in welfare and a slow death sentence was imposed on many of our people. That is why our young people act strange. "Oh, we'll get 'soosi' (social allowance)," they say. "We'll celebrate. The older people will all go to bingo hall tonight." Social allowance has really done harm to our people. This type of money does not make a person rich. All it does is provide a little bit of food money and the rest is spent on non-essentials. Not very many want to work. Our hands are all soft.

Who grows their own crops today? White farmers are working all the fields. Why aren't the children being taught things like growing crops and vegetables and raising cattle? All they're learning is the computers. This is not going to help them if there is a disaster.

Disasters are happening now. Look at all the earthquakes and the planes going down. We are being punished by the Creator. We're very lucky that we have not experienced the tornadoes or earthquakes here on our reserve.

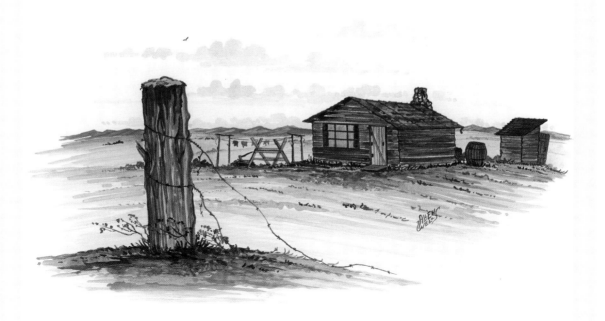

Omahksiko'ksstaotsimaiksi – Big Corner Post Clan

AAMOSTSKAI AISSKSINI'PI—VALUES WE THINK ABOUT

CULTURAL BACKGROUND INFORMATION

- Talk to your children all the time.
- Look after your things.
- Listen to your parents, your grandparents.
- Do not fight with others.
- Look after your horse.
- Respect prayer.
- Use your common sense.
- Respect the culture of our people.
- Respect the old people, share something you have with them, help them in any way you can.
- Observe nature and respect the animals and the earth.
- Remember you are a part of nature, not above it.
- Respect the knowledge of elders and learn the proper way to ask for help.
- Honour the memory of your parents, grandparents and elders.
- Be tolerant of the beliefs of others, do not make fun of them.
- Be respectful to your teachers.
- Share and be hospitable.
- Do not put too much value in material possessions.
- Do not expect payment for doing good.
- Have compassion for others.
- Be sincere in your relations with others.
- Remember that you have a responsibility for the people of the future.
- Love one another.
- Pray for simple things, gentle things.
- Never give up, always complete a task.
- Work not to finish quickly but to finish well.
- Learn as many good and useful skills as you can.
- Keep yourself busy.
- Learn about plants.
- Learn the signs of nature.
- Be prepared for anything.
- Do not be afraid to learn about spirituality.
- Learn about our people's history.
- Learn your family's history.
- Listen to your parents and grandparents so that you will know what to do in the future.
- Learn from your mistakes.
- Face hardships and challenges head on, never give up.
- You will not get something good by doing bad.
- You will have good luck if you do good things.

Geography

Original Location

The truth about our original location is shrouded in the mists of time. Without the luxury of books and written history, it is difficult to determine where our original location was. Not being able to pinpoint dates is one of the shortcomings of an oral history.

Anthropologists and other social scientists have determined that we were originally a woodland tribe. If this is true then we were probably originally located somewhere in what is now eastern Canada (probably western Ontario or eastern Manitoba).

Through some force, which created a domino effect once it got started, some original eastern tribes were pushed westward. Niitsitapi was one of these tribes. This was when Kainai, Siksika and Piikani were still one tribe.

Eventually, our domain became what it was when contact occurred around the 1730s. Our northern boundary was the North Saskatchewan River. In the east it was the Cypress Hills. To the south it was the Missouri River, and in the west it was the Rocky Mountains. When our grandfathers made treaty in 1877, the resulting boundaries of our separate reserves were greatly reduced.

At the Treaty 7 signing held at Blackfoot Crossing in 1877, our grandfathers signed a treaty in good faith, believing that what they agreed to in words was what was stated in the text of the treaty. They believed that they were signing a peace treaty which would curtail intrusion into Niitsitapi territory.

Mode of Travel

Prior to the acquisition of the horse after 1735, the mode of travel of Niitsitapi was by foot (pedestrian). The people who lived in this period are referred to as Iimitaota'si or "those who used the dog as a horse." This was literally true since the dog was used as a beast of burden. It was used for hauling possessions from place to place. Because of their limited hauling capacity, families were either forced to limit their possessions or, if they had more stuff, to carry these themselves.

Within a short period of time following the acquisition of the horse, Niitsitapi society changed radically. Travel was not only easier, but distances could be covered faster. The people came into contact with distant tribes and there was more conflict with other tribes. Because horse ownership was so prized, there was a lot of horse thieving between tribes of the plains.

Niitsitapii society was greatly altered by the arrival of the horse. As if they had always had the horse, Niitsitapii men and boys became expert horsemen in no time. Because the horse was a bigger animal than the dog, it became the beast of burden. This meant that a man could have a bigger lodge and eventually more than one wife.

In fact, wealth and prestige came with horse ownership. The more horses a man had, the more he could share with members of his clan. Aahsitapiisini and kimmapiipitsini were two values which became more emphasized.

Environmental Effects

The prairie environment naturally had a great influence on Niitsitapii life. The prairie was the home of iinii (buffalo), which roamed its vast area freely. This animal was like a superstore to Niitsitapi because it provided all the essentials of life. It was the chief source for food. The meat and the various organs as well as the blood were all consumed.

The hide was worn as a robe, used as bedding, or was sewn together with other hides and put over a wooden structure. This became the niitoyis (tipi). Some of the bones and organs became utensils or containers. Not much waste occurred when a buffalo was killed by Niitsitapii.

After the arrival of the horse and mobility was greatly enhanced, Niitsitapii freely roamed the vast prairie. Contact was made with more tribes, both friendly and adversarial. The former oftentimes accompanied trade for items previously unknown and unfamiliar.

With more property and more mobility, the family size was extended. Men took more wives out of necessity. These wives were primarily needed to help move a lodge and its furnishings at short notice.

KAINAISSKSAHKOYI

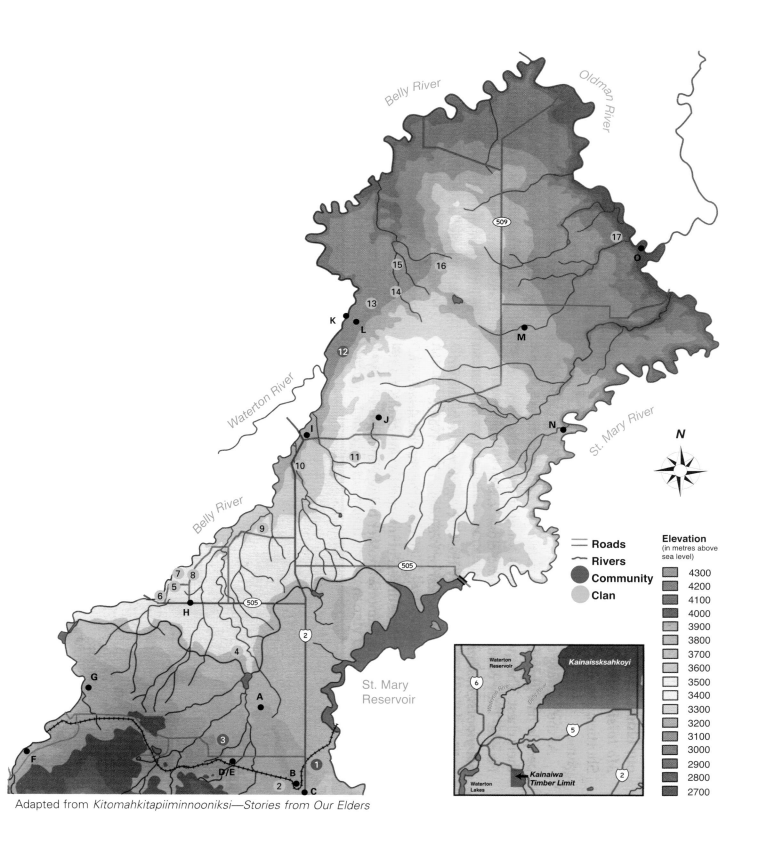

Adapted from *Kitomahkitapiiminnooniksi—Stories from Our Elders*

LEGEND

A. Kainai Board of Education
   - *Kainai* High School
   - *Tatsikiisaapo'p* Middle School
   - Red Crow Community College
   - *Sikaiipisstsiitaissksinima'tstohkio'pi*–St. Mary's Roman Catholic Indian Residential School (1926–1950s)
B. *Itaisokinakio'pi*–Blood Indian Hospital
C. *Aakaohkiimiiksi*–Cardston
D. *Sa'ksisoka'simiitaissksinima'tstohkio'pi*–St. Paul's Anglican Indian Residental School (1924–1950s)
E. St. Paul's Treatment Center
F. *Aakaomissko*–Creek of Many Fish
G. *Iitsiksikkihkiniooyoo'pi*–Where the Bald Eagles Nest
H. *Aahsaopi* Elementary School
I. *Tatsikiitapiwa*–Standoff
Former site of:
   - *Sikaipistsiitaissksinima'tstohkio'pi*–Roman Catholic Mission (1898–1926)
   - *Iikaitaisokinakio'p*–Roman Catholic Mission Hospital (1890s–1926)
   - *Iikaitaisttsinao'p*–Former Ration House
Present site of:
   - *Iitonnio'pi*–Shot Both Sides Administration
   - *Saipoyi* Elementary School
   - *I'nakitaisokinakio'p*–Health Center
   - Kainai Continuing Care Center
   - Human Resources Building
   - Blood Tribe Police Department
   - Kainai Community Corrections
J. *Mookowansin*–Belly Buttes:
   Location of annual traditional social and spiritual gathering
K. *Omahksini*–Big Island (location of first Anglican Residential School)
L. *Iikaitonnio'pi*–Old Agency
M. *Makiinimaa*–Blood Tribe Agricultural Project
N. *Kainaisikoohkotok*–Black Horse Mines
O. *Iitoka'poyi'nitspi*–site of *Iitoka'poyi'nitspi* Fort Whoop-Up "Where many people died"

CLANS AND COMMUNITIES OF THE KAINAI NATION

1. *Niipokskaitapiiksi*
2. *I'siisoka'simiiksi*
3. *Spikskoitapiiksi*
4. *Aakaipokaiksi* and later *I'naksiiksi*
5. *Mamioyiiksi*
6. *Sikohkitsimiiksi*
7. *Isskssiinaisimiiksi*
8. *Omahksiko'ksstao'tsimaiksi*
9. *Pottstakiiksi* and later *Aisspahkomiiksi*
10. *Ni'taitsskaiksi*
11. *Ipakinamaiksi*
12. *Sooyiootsipisskoitapiiksi*
13. *Aakaiksamaiksi*
14. *Mo'toisikskiiksi*
15. *Mo'toikkakssiiksi*
16. *Mo'toisspitaiksi*
17. *Namoopisiiksi*